Haraka, Haraka ...
Look before you leap

YOUTH AT THE CROSSROAD
OF CUSTOM AND MODERNITY

Edited by
Magdalena K. Rwebangira
and
Rita Liljeström

Nordiska Afrikainstitutet, 1998

This book is published with support from Sida, through its Department for Research Cooperation (SAREC).

Indexing terms
Sociology
Youth
Gender
Sexuality
Pregnancy
Marriage
Child welfare
Education
Family law
Customary law
Tanzania

Cover: Adriaan Honcoop

Cover photo: Rita Liljeström

Map: Mr. Mathias Ngowi, Cartographic Unit, Department of Geography, University of Dar es Salaam

Copyediting: Peter Colenbrander

ISBN 91-7106-429-X

Printed in Sweden by Elanders Gotab, Stockholm 1998

Contents

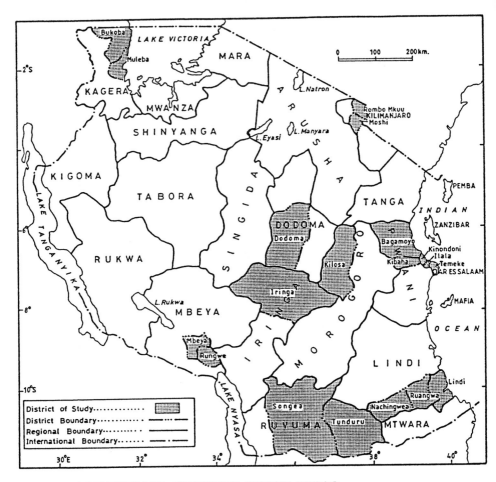

MAP OF TANZANIA SHOWING STUDY AREAS

Chapter 2
Mbeya Region
(Mbeya Town in Mbeya District
Tukuyu Town in Rungwe
District)

Chapter 3
Lindi Region
(Ruangwa and Nachingwea
District)

Chapter 4
Dodoma Region
(Simba Chunzachi Division
in Dodoma District)
Ruvuma Region
(Mbesa Village in Nalasi Ward,
Tunduru District)

Chapter 5
Dar es Salaam Region
(Manzese Ward in Kinondoni
District)
Mbeya Region

(Mwanjelwa Ward in Mbeya
District)

Chapter 6
Kilimanjaro Region
(Keni Aleni in Rombo District)
Morogoro Region
(Gairo Ward in Kilosa District)

Chapter 7
Dar es Salaam Region
(Bunju Ward in Kinondoni District)
Pwani/Coast Region
Kibaha and Bagamoyo Districts
Kagera Region
(Kishanje Ward in Bukoba
District)
(Buganguzi Ward in Muleba
District)

Chapter 8
Dar es Salaam Region
(Masasani, Masaki, Kunduchi,
Namanga and Oysterbay in

Kinondoni District)
Kigamboni in Temeke District
Ruvuma Region
(Songe Town in Songea District)

Chapter 9
Dar es Salaam Region
(Mnazi Mmoja, Ferry Mkunguni
in Ilala District)
(Tandika in Temeke District)
Morogoro Region
(Morogoro Town in Morogoro
District)

Chapter 10
Dar es Salaam Region
(Temeke in Temeke District)
Iringa Region
(Iringa Town in Iringa District)
Mbeya Region
(Mbeya Town in Mbeya District)
Kilimanjaro Region
(Moshi in Moshi District)

Preface

Haraka, Haraka is, like the title of our first book, *Chelewa, Chelewa*, de-rived from a Kiswahili proverb: *Haraka, Haraka, Haina Baraka*. This means "Rushed action has no blessing", or *Look before you leap*. In the former book we criticized the delays in delivering reproductive health information and services to teenage girls. The studies in *Haraka, Haraka* lament the rapid disintegration of family values and the com-munity's relinquishment of its common responsibility to nurture ado-lescents and groom them as accountable adults. The modern state has so far not managed to fill the vacuum left by abandoned rituals and symbols that accompanied and instilled meaning into the reproduc-tive cycle.

The Teenage Girls' Reproductive Health Study Group was estab-lished in 1988–89. It is based at the University of Dar es Salaam. The group is the brainchild of two of the earliest women's organizations at the university's main campus, the Women's Research and Documen-tation Project (WRDP) and the Institute of Development Studies Women's Study Group (IDS-WSG). Professor Rita Liljeström from Gothenburg University, Sweden, wrote to the two women's groups on behalf of the Swedish Agency for Research Cooperation with Devel-oping Countries (SAREC), to inquire about our interest in studying reproductive health issues from a social science perspective. When we met Rita Liljeström in Dar es Salaam, we told her about our particular interest in teenage girls. At the first meeting with Professor Rita, as she is affectionately known to the group, the Teenage Girls' Repro-ductive Health Study Group was formed. It is made up of ten women from the two women's groups. We wrote abstracts and applications. When Professor Rita next visited Dar es Salaam, there were outlines for ten studies. Those studies were included in *Chelewa, Chelewa. The Dilemma of Teenage Girls*.

Our group is professionally diverse and multidisciplinary. Three of its members are academics at the University of Dar es Salaam. We include an educationalist, a lexicographer, a primary school teacher, an environmentalist cultural geographer, an administrator, an editor, a youth counsellor, and a private legal practitioner. This diversity has been one of our greatest resources and has enriched our discussions.

Our ethnic and regional origins differ. Whereas I come from Bukoba district in Kagera, Juliana Mzira and Alice Rugumyamheto hail from Same in Kilimanjaro. Mary Shuma from Moshi is also from Kilimanjaro region. Zubeida Tumbo-Masabo, Mary Ntukula and Betty Komba-Malekela are from the South. Rosalia Katapa comes from Tukuyu in Mbeya region, and Grace Puja is from Singida region. Usually, we started our education at missionary schools. The group has different religious beliefs: some are Christians, some Muslims, and others adhere to old African beliefs or are secularized.

Two members of the group did not contribute to Haraka, Haraka, as they are taking advantage of opportunities provided by SAREC. Betty Komba-Malekela is pursuing studies in Britain, and Grace Puja is doing her Ph.D. in Canada.

It is now ten years since Professor Rita raised the study idea with our groups and nine years since we began to work together. Besides the three sets of studies we have undertaken, the most remarkable development in the group is the bonding among its members. We have become a family, participating in each other's funerals, weddings, religious ceremonies, and joining hands to share in pains and joys. After years of studying and discussing teenagers, we have together watched most of our own children become teenager. Consequently, we have had the often rare opportunity in modern society to discuss and share experiences of the growing pains of our teenage children among ourselves as colleagues.

As all our research work is done part-time, we have struggled together to learn, and have encouraged each other to fit it in with our other schedules. The knowledge gained from the studies over the years has given us a deeper insight into the developmental and reproductive rights issues facing our country, our communities, ourselves as parents, and especially the teenagers of Tanzania. We consider the time spent on this work to have been well spent.

The history of women's groups at the University of Dar es Salaam is rather remarkable. They date back a long way to the awakening of the women's movements in Tanzania. Just before the Third United Nations World Conference in Nairobi 1985, the IDS's Women's Study Group was formed as part and parcel of the Institute of Development Studies of the university. This study group consists of both academic and non-academic members of staff in the institute as well as women who are outside the university but interested in working together to study women's issues. In 1982, another group, not affiliated to any institution, was established under the name of the Women's Research and Documentation Project. Like the Womens' Study Group it comprised both academic and non-academic members. The interaction between academics and field operators added to the richness of the two groups. The groups helped to raise gender issues, do research, and produce documentation through seminars, the documentation centre, and consultancy services. Both of these groups have extended their original roles and they now even provide outreach services.

Not surprisingly, the 1990s saw a strong women's movement on campus with the formation of Women in Education (WED) in 1989, and Tanzania Women's Science and Technology (TAWOSTE) in 1992. The groups are voluntary but some activities, particularly research and equipment acquisition, are externally funded, while the university provides office accommodation and some basic furniture. It was probably partly due to the number of these groups that SAREC, the main donor to their research activities, recently required the gender groups to take care of their own administration of funds through the newly established Gender Management Committee (GMC). All gender study groups on campus are represented, except the Teenage Girls' Reproductive Health Study Group, which is not a formal group. However, with shrinking resources for research, the gender groups on campus now face an insecure future. Authorities have decided that all research funds coming through the university shall be allocated on a competitive basis and not through gender groups. Furthermore, the awarding of research funds to non-academic researchers is not viewed favourably, given that resources for research are scant because of ongoing economic reforms.

The group has enjoyed constructive discussions and support from the resource team, whose members have been more and more involved in the issues over the years. The first workshop concerning *Haraka, Haraka* was held at the Elimu na Malezi ya Ujana (EMAU) premises in Upanga, Dar es Salaam, in April 1996. Present were Mr. M. Tuguta, Ministry of Education and Culture, Mr. Cletus Mkai, Bureau of Statistics, Professor Ernest Urassa, Muhimbili University College of Health Science, and the sociologist, Ms. Rose Mwaipopo-Ako, University of Dar es Salaam. Professor Edmund Dahlström joined his wife, Professor Rita, at the workshop. By 1996, these two had retired as professors of sociology. The authors presented their chapters and the participants criticized and commented on them.

In October 1996, Professor Ernest Urassa, Mrs. Mary Machuve, Ministry of Education and Culture (who replaced Mr. Tuguta who was pursuing Ph.D. studies), Mrs. Tuli Kassimoto, Ministry of Community Development, Women's Affairs, and Children, and the sociologist, Dr. Patrick Masanja, Dar es Salaam University, joined us at Gogo Hotel in Bagamoyo to discuss the framework of the first chapter and to devote attention to progress reports from our third set of studies.

We want to express our thanks to the Swedish Agency for Research Cooperation with Developing Countries (SAREC) and the Swedish International Development Cooperation Agency (Sida) for unwavering support for our activities. We are also grateful to the support we have enjoined to date from the Universities of Gothenburg and Dar es Salaam, which have provided a unique opportunity for multidisciplinary or multiprofessional studies, cooperation, and friendship. This list would not be complete without emphasizing our resource persons, who have always been willing to accommodate us. Mr. Cletus Mkai and Ms. Rose Mwaipopo-Ako are particularly acknowledged for providing basic data for the first chapter of *Haraka, Haraka*. However, we owe most to our families for their support and patience throughout the research and writing exercises and the emotional strains that accompany them, particularly when they have to be combined with other work, as was the case here.

Magdalena K. Rwebangira

Chapter 1
Cultural Conflicts and Ambiguities

*Rita Liljeström, Patrick Masanja, Magdalena K. Rwebangira,
and Ernest J.N. Urassa*

Modern law versus customary law

Tanzania as a nation state came into being on 9 December 1961 when
Tanganyika attained its independence from Britain. Until then, the
more than 120 communities making up Tanganyika were tribal group-
ings characterized by different levels of centralized or decentralized
authority and were mostly regulated by traditional customs. Colonial
rulers introduced new laws which operated side by side with the customary laws of the local communities. Among these new laws were,
*the Interpretation and General Clauses Act, Indian Acts (and Application),
Subordinate Courts Ordinance, the Children and Young Person's Ordinance, Adoption Ordinance, the Penal Code,* and *the Witchcraft Ordinance.*
These laws pertained to commerce and trade, criminal law administration and the centralization of government. Furthermore, there
colonial power acceded to a number of international treaties which
later applied to independent Tanzania. Most of these laws were be-
queathed to the independent state, which also made its own state
laws.

What did this mean for local governments and their traditional
customs? Probably the most significant impact of these changes for
local people was that some of their customs were outlawed. The
power of chiefs was limited under the British colonial government
policy of indirect rule, chiefly jurisdiction in criminal matters was
ended and the cash economy, with its vagaries of taxation and
integration into the international capitalist system, was introduced.

The postindependence government has largely built on the work
of the colonial state. However, it did away with the indirect rule of the
British colonial government, and sought to modernize entire communities within its borders under uniform laws enforced by centralized
state machinery. This modernizing mission has seen the passing of

laws such as the codification of customary law in 1963, the *Law of Marriage Act* 1971 and the *Education Act* 1978. All of these have changed local gender relations and, particularly, relations between elders and young people.

The period from independence to the mid-1970s saw the expansion of the role of the state. *Ujamaa*, Tanzania's brand of socialism based on communal production and distribution, brought new perspectives and the hope of rural development to a poor country. The state took the leading role, reducing the people's role to that of spectators and followers (Havnevik, 1993). Needless to say, despite obvious good intentions and some success for national unity, the state's economic policy was a failure. This failure forced the Tanzanian leadership to give in to the conditions of international institutions such as the International Monetary Fund and the World Bank. The Structural Adjustment Programme (SAP) and Economic Structural Adjustment Programme (ESAP) were among those conditions. One far-reaching characteristic of these programmes has been the call on the state to reduce its role in the social and economic life of the nation. This, coupled with a deteriorating national economy and increased dependency on external financing, has meant a reduction of state funding on education, health services, and the general social sector. Consequently, the modern health and education services introduced in the 1960s and 1970s have suffered seriously from a want of care and maintenance.

As a result the morale of teachers has been low in both rural and urban areas. Many schools have no desks and lack adequate educational material such as textbooks and exercise books, not to mention the technical equipment necessary for scientific experiments in laboratories. Similarly, the modern health facilities (concentrated in urban centres) have suffered from a lack of drugs and trained personnel. As a result, the modernization campaign, which encouraged people to enrol children in schools and to abandon traditional healers and birth attendants, now sounds hollow in the face of malfunctional modern facilities. Furthermore, as with many poor African nations, the Tanzanian state's ability to meet its economic obligations has eroded rapidly.

These trends have raised doubts as to whether the African nation state as we know it is withering away and, if so, what implications this will have for the younger generation? Should they look to the state to enforce the modern laws or should they settle for the old and sometimes repressive order. Is the state capable of blending viable elements of the older order and suppressing obscurantists ones while promoting desirable change? The question is where is the old order and whether we can identify it.

In the traditional village, events that cannot be explained are seen as expressions of witchcraft, and popular anxieties are somewhat held in balance by such means. At the religious level, major events are associated either with the works of God or the devil and human minds are kept in balance by such beliefs. Differences in knowledge and understanding, in social and economic assets, in worldviews and aspirations, in the perception of modernity and what it can offer, in the rate at which traditional life collapses and the demands of modernity assert themselves, result in confusion, conflict and ambiguity. These are the main topics addressed by the authors of this book based on their field research in villages and towns in Tanzania. Our themes range from the changing roles of family members, to the collapse of customary initiation, to the inadequacy of the modern educational system, to customary versus modern family formation procedures, to the effects of Islam, Christian and old African religious values and so on. The chapters enlarge on aspects of the issues previously discussed in *Chelewa, Chelewa* (1994) and seeks to reveal the complexities involved.

When we the Teenage Reproductive Health Study Group conducted our first set of studies, we focused on the plight of teenage girls. In initiating a second set of studies we became aware of the need to expand our scope to embrace the social institutions that regulate reproduction; initiation into adulthood, marriage, and parental obligations. In order to understand institutional change over time, Rosalia S. Katapa and Mary Shuma have interviewed women and men of different generations. Moreover, we have included men, potential boyfriends, husbands, or runaway fathers in half the studies. In some of these men are the main characters.

The book begins with studies of changes in the marital patterns of the patrilineal Nyakusa and the matrilineal Wamwera. Rosalia S. Katapa calls her study "Nyakusa Teenage Sexuality—Past and Present". We have all tried to reach a closer understanding of sub-Saharan concepts of "sexuality". Katapa's topic is transformation of gender and marriage. Yet she notes that although she has been thinking about the meaning of sexuality for a long time, it has escaped her. Nevertheless, she ends by calling her study "Nyakusa Teenage Sexuality—Past and Present", arguing that "this is how I understand sexuality." In a sense, she gets to the hearth of the matter.

What are sexual relations?

In *The History of Sexuality* (1978), Michel Foucault distinguishes between two kinds of deployment that sex relations give rise to in societies. The first is known as *deployment of alliance*

> ... a system of marriage, of fixation and development of kinship ties, of transmission of names and possessions. This deployment of alliance, with the mechanisms of constraint that ensured its existence and the complex knowledge it often required, lost some of its importance as economic processes and political structures could no longer rely on it. ... Particularly from the eighteenth century onward, Western societies created and deployed a new apparatus which was superimposed on the previous one, and which, without completely supplanting the latter, helped to reduce its importance (p. 106).

> The second type, *deployment of sexuality*, also "connects up with the circuit of sexual partners, but in a completely different way. The two systems can be contrasted term by term" (p. 106). The *deployment of alliance* is built around a system of rules defining the permitted and forbidden, the licit and illicit. One of its chief objectives is to reproduce the interplay of relations and maintain the law that governs them: what is pertinent is the link between partners and definite statuses. The *deployment of alliance* is firmly tied to the economy because of the role it can play in the transmission or circulation of wealth. Hence, here the important phase concerns reproduction.

> On the other hand, *deployment of sexuality* operates according to mobile, manifold, and contingent techniques of power. It engenders a continual extension of areas and forms of control. The *deployment of sexuality* is concerned with the sensations of body, the quality of pleasures, and the nature of impressions. It is linked to the economy through numerous and subtle relays, the main one of which is the body—the body that produces and consumes. It is not governed by reproduction; it is body-centred. It has been linked from the outset with an intensification of the body; with its exploitation as an object of knowledge and an element in relations of power (p. 107).

> According to Foucault, there has been "a gradual progression away from the problematic of the relations toward a problematic of the 'flesh', that is, of the body, sensation, the nature of pleasure. ... 'Sexuality' was taking shape, born of a technology of power that was originally focused on alliance. Since then, it has not ceased to operate in conjunction with a system of alliance on which it has depended for support" (p. 108).

> The historical transition from sex for reproduction to sex for pleasure, means a transition from control by religion to control by science, from morality to rationality, followed by a transfer of power from the church to the clinic. This transition has evolved since the seventeenth century. Throughout the nineteenth century sex was incorporated into two very distinct orders of knowledge: on the one hand, comprehension of a biology of reproduction and on the other, a medicine of sexuality, each of them conforming to very different rules. There was no real exchange between them. They were kept apart (pp. 54–5).

The discursive construction of something called "sexuality" is embedded in Western social history and cultural particularities. When the Western mores and diagnoses were later imposed on sub-Saharan peoples by missionaries and medical doctors, they were introduced either as religious morality and decency, or as health issues within the current frame of sexual and reproductive health and fertility control. To the receivers "sexuality" remained a shallow modern concept. While everyone pretends to understand what it refers to, the clinical concept did not correspond to local people's understanding of their world. This did not disturb either those who founded churches or those who built hospitals, as they believed in the universality of their God and their Knowledge.

In an effort to contain maternal and infant mortality, the spread of STDs and HIV/AIDS, and population growth, other professions and practitioners have been mobilized to help solve problems which have expanded beyond the field of health and medicine. One ought to remember that the concept "sexuality" was established in Europe in the process of the medicalization of the body, and there did not exist in African cosmologies a particular concept of "sexuality" focused on gender and procreation.

Among the Sukuma-Nyamwezi the very expressions for woman and man convey a message of reproductive power. The words for feminine and masculine refer to the genitals of the sexes. Women and men represent human fecundity. A man who has fathered many children is a "true" man , and a women of proven fecundity is a "true" woman. Since human fertility is always under threat, there is always much preoccupation among women and men to safeguard this attribute, and to restore it through rituals and medical devices (Brandström, 1990).

"Sexuality" illuminates the dangers of using European terms and expressions uncritically when addressing non-European cultures and

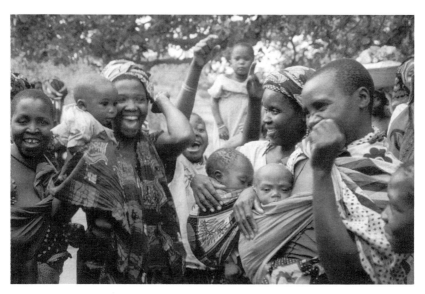

Women and men represent human fecundity.   (Photo Rita Liljeström)
A woman of proven fecundity is a "true" woman.

experiences. "The language which has aided the European imperial project is loaded with generalized terms which do not necessarily have common meaning", warns Amadiume (1997). We have participated in several workshops designed for research and other interventions. After days of discussion, someone usually has the courage to say, "I do not understand what you really mean by sexuality." Then other African participants usually confirm this general confusion. There must be something more to it than the bare sexual act itself. How do people think about it? Is there some superior and advanced modern meaning attached to it? This seemingly elusive meaning is what often confuses African participants. In many ways, sexuality and "sexual behaviour" are discussed without regard to the lack of common cultural frames. The Western claim of universal progress and competence seems to have contributed to an African tendency to turn away from indigenous models of gender, potence, and fertility.

John Mbiti (1969) has the following to say about sex in African societies

> In African societies sex is not used for biological purposes alone. It has also religious and social uses. For procreation and pleasure, sex plays an obvious and important role. ... There are African peoples among whom rituals are solemnly opened and concluded with actual or symbolic sex-

ual intercourse between husband and wife or other officiating persons. This is like a solemn seal or signature, where sex is used in and as a sacred action, as a "sacrament" signifying inward spiritual values ...

There are areas where sex is used as an expression of hospitality. This means that when a man visits another, the custom is for the host to give his wife (or daughter or sister) to the guest so that the two can sleep together. In other societies, the brothers have rights to the wives of their brothers (remembering here that a person has hundreds of brothers and their wives are "potentially" his wives as well). Where the age-group system is taken very seriously, like among the Maasai, members of one group who were initiated in the same batch, are entitled to have sexual relations with the other fellow members. In cases where the husband is forced by circumstances to live away from his wife, it may also be arranged by the individuals concerned, and with the passive understanding of the community, that a friend (normally of the "brother" relationship) may go to his wife and have sexual intercourse with her as may be convenient, partly to satisfy her sexual urge and thus preventing her from going about with anybody, and partly to fertilize her and raise children to the absent "father". The same arrangements are made where the husband is either too young, impotent or sterile. All these are acceptable uses of sex; but how far they are actually observed in real life one cannot say without a proper study of the subject (pp. 146–7).

Obviously, Mbiti describes an ideal type of *deployment of alliance* in an African cultural context. It was a challenge to our team to explore old ethnic orders in an attempt to understand what has changed and what remains, and how changes have upset the smooth relationships within communities. The *old deployments of alliance* were shaken and eroding due to influences from outside: first the Christian message of sin and European concepts of decency; then, the "modernization of sex", which turned from considering the bonds of the social body to the biological body, from a sacred drama to a stage of risky pleasures.

Reform and erosion of previous orders

The Nyakusa were once a patriarchal society with a marked male age-group organization. In fact, one can speak of age segregation among men. Elderly men were unwilling to contribute to the bridewealth of their sons because they competed with them for young wives. Consequently, the marital age among women was low, while men had to wait for a long time. To overcome obstacles to marriage, several solutions were at hand. Rosalia S. Katapa discusses methods that were used in the past to get wives: by inheritance, by seizing or snatching a wife, by elopement, and by rape. It is no surprise to learn that the Nyakusa attached great significance to virginity.

Mary Shuma provides a vivid picture in her "The Erosion of the Matrilineal Order of the Wamwera". Here the roles of husband and father were secondary to those of the maternal uncle and brother. Probably, the tension between maternal and paternal priorities, men being torn between their sisters and wives, or more precisely, between the children of their sisters and the children of their wives, is the fragile link in the matrilineal chain.

While Nyakusa and Wamwera were markedly different in the way they organized gender and marriage in the past, there are certain similarities in their current situation. In both cases, people are troubled by teenage pregnancies out-of-wedlock and men's unwillingness to marry. In both societies, the maternal grandparents take care of their unmarried daughters' children. Divorces have become more common. Both chapters point to the impact of education, new roads to remote villages, increased contacts with foreigners, and tribal inter-marriage.

The mixed blessings of education

For Nyakusa girls, education has meant an end to arranged marriages and virginity controls. Furthermore, education has meant later marriages and women being less dependent on their husbands. Schooling introduces changes in the lifecycle of individuals. As noted, the age of marriage rises. For example, the *Tanzania Demographic and Health Survey* of 1991/92 reveals that the median age of first marriage varied with educational attainment:

Level of education	Median age of first marriage
no education	16.7 years
completed primary school	19.9 years
secondary and higher education	23.0 years

Source: *Tanzania Demographic and Health Survey*, p. 55.

Delay in marriage, however, does not preclude sexual activity:

Per cent of those who have had sexual intercourse by age	
23 per cent	15 years
65 per cent	18 years
83 per cent	20 years

Source: *Tanzania Demographic and Health Survey*, p. 56.

In relation to educational background of women aged 25 to 49, the median age at first intercourse was as follows:

Median age at first intercourse
15 years for those with no education
16.3 years for those with incomplete primary school
18 years with completed primary education
20.4 years for those with secondary and higher education

Source: *Tanzania Demographic and Health Survey*, p. 57.

According to the same source, 71.8 per cent of teenage girls in the 15 to 19 age category were never married (p. 51). The *Tanzania Knowledge, Attitudes and Practices Survey* of 1994 indicates that "half the women of Tanzania get married before age eighteen" (p. 52) and that "27 per cent of currently married women are in polygynous unions" (abstracted from Table 5.2 of *Tanzania Demographic and Health Survey* 1991/92).

The school system has exposed communities to new cultures through numeracy and literacy, and it has introduced changes in life-cycles, thus affecting both customary initiation rites and the age of marriage. While the educational system has opened avenues to the labour market for those who manage to reach its higher levels, the same educational system leaves adolescents unprepared when it comes to human reproduction and gender. The youth is thus exposed and disarmed. Education has evidently not been able to replace customary initiation and upbringing, at least not in many rural communities. Neither has it had the imaginativeness to look for integration between some customs and modern instruction. Initiations for girls and boys (*unyago* and *jando*) are still a feature of growing up among, for example, the Wamwera and Wagogo people. Among Wamwera the conflicting interest between modern education and customary initiation (including a period of seclusion) has led to initiation at lower ages and of shorter duration. This, among other things, seems to have undermined its meaning.

This timing of events in the lifecycle gives rise to tensions and problems. Many teenagers are exposed to and become conscious of issues of sexuality at a time when schooling does not allow them to get married and when dominant values discourage premarital relations. Furthermore, the content and message of customary initiation does not satisfy youth who have some knowledge of biology, for example. Initiation for a traditional society is losing its context and relevance in a modernizing society. On the other hand, the modern educational system is either not prepared or is prevented from touching on the topic and from teaching safe sexuality and pregnancy prevention.

Thus, while customary initiation is losing its context, the modern educational system remains ill-equipped to prepare the young for adulthood. This may not be true for the three R's perhaps, but it is so concerning sexual and reproductive relationships. Instruction in these topics remains unorganized in urban areas and relies on out-of-context customary practices in rural communities. While the school hesitates to provide new medical devices for fertility control, it is even less prepared to discuss contradictions between sacred clan values and the rational and individualized values of modern education.

The sociologist Anthony Giddens (1991), while reflecting on modernity in the West, writes about *rites de passage* in a way which is also valid for Africa:

> ... rites de passage are relatively lacking in modern societies in respect of basic transitions, including the beginning and end of life. Most such discussions emphasise that, without ordered ritual and collective involvement, individuals are left without structured ways of coping with the tensions and anxieties involved. Communal rites provide a focus of group solidarity at major transitions as well as allocating definite tasks for those involved ...

> However, something more profound is lost together with traditional forms and ritual. *Rites de passage* place those concerned in touch with wider cosmic forces, relating individual life to more encompassing existential issues. Traditional ritual, as well as religious belief, connected individual action to moral frameworks and to elemental questions about human existence. The loss of ritual is also a loss of involvement in such frameworks, however ambiguously they might have been experienced and however much they were bound up with traditional religious discourse (p. 204).

Current contradictions and ambiguities

The plight of teenage girls in different communities in Tanzania is shaped by forces of change which are both national and global. These forces mould the social contexts of teenagers. This social and cultural context contains paradoxes, conflicts, ambiguities, and a host of problems mixed with prospects and possibilities that generate hope for the future.

"Training by Symbolism and Imagery: The Case of Wagogo and Wayao" by Zubeida Tumbo-Masabo explores initiation rites in a matrilineal and a patrilineal village. Both tribes practise a set of rites of passage that continually instruct the individual at puberty, menarche, before marriage, and before childbirth. The secrecy that surrounds the rites renders the study of them difficult. The two tribes see themselves as being confronted by modern interventions: a school system that spoils children and undermines the norms of the community, and hence, encourages out-of-wedlock pregnancies. Moreover, the Wagogo, who use female circumcision, are targeted by a campaign against circumcision that is led by educated women. Local women blame the government for lack of respect for traditions while bluntly denying any negative effects of the customs. It is a rural–urban conflict, one of many between people on the periphery and at the centre.

Another source of cultural ambivalence is the religious pluralism one finds in different parts of Tanzania. Customary religious beliefs and values coexist with those of Christianity and Islam. For followers of different religions, there are tensions in terms of what tenets to adhere to regarding premarital sex, extramarital relationships, monogamy and polygamy, female circumcision, etc. These are real challenges that adults and teenagers have to contend with in terms of moral attitudes towards gender relations. On such existential issues as the way in which we choose to bring up children, relate to marriage, and our attitudes towards illness and death, customary values underlie many practices of individuals and families, even though these values are contested by modernity and other religious teachings. Even non-adherents of Islam and Christianity are affected by cultural influences arising from these religions and from other communities within and outside Tanzania. Impressions from our fieldwork suggest that people combine elements from different religions in quite free and flexible ways.

Recurrent ambiguities and contradictions need to be understood in light of the social and political history of the country. Two recent books explain and elaborate two modes of power originating in the colonial period (Mamdani, 1996; Reader, 1997).

The colonial state used two complementary modes of controlling "natives" in the early colonial period. Direct rule was the form of urban civil power, whereas indirect rule signified a rural tribal authority. The latter aimed at incorporating natives into a state-enforced customary order (Mamdani, 1996).

Every African colony had two legal systems, one modern and one customary. The claim to legitimacy of customary law was that it was a tribal law, and of customary authorities that they were tribal authorities administering tribal law. Tribalism was the essential form of colonial rule. The tribes, customs, and the customary law were defined or interpreted in the interests of the colonial state.

The seat of customary power in rural areas was the local state, the district. The local-state functionary was called the chief. Behind the administrative justice and coercion that were the sum of his authority, lay a regime of extra-economic coercion, a regime that broke life down into a whole range of compulsory activities: forced labour, forced crops, forced sales, forced contributions, and forced removals. The local state was organized as an ethnic power to enforce customs on tribespeople. Needless to say, customs and customary law were defined and interpreted in the interest of the colonial state. Customary law consolidated the non-customary power of the chiefs. Previously autonomous domains like the household, age-groups, and gender associations now fell within the scope of chiefly power.

What did the tribes look like at the time of the introduction of customary law? According to Mamdani, there was seldom a clear separation of tribes or even a homogeneous internal culture in those times of great change and tension. The tendency was for more or less mixing of tribes and internal differentiation that allowed for varied and even conflicting practices within the same tribe. Not only were the boundaries blurred, there was often little that was traditional about the tribal boundaries that were drawn by the colonial administration.

Tribal culture was highly textured and elastic, and strangers were often present. Where status and wealth accrued to a household, kin group or a community, they could attract dependants or followers, "strangers" who were welcomed as wives, clients, "blood brothers", settlers or disciples because they enhanced the prestige and often the labour force of the head of the group. As a result, communities were more often than not multiethnic. In such a context, to identify community with tribe was to sow the seeds of much tension. With the state-enforced notion of custom, the tendency was to homogenize and flatten cultural diversity within the tribe in favour of an official version of "tribe".

While customary law has always taken contemporary assessment into account in its judgments, once a particular set of interpretations was codified, colonial law became rigid and unable to reflect change. The customary law applied to Native Authorities condemned a rural community "to live in a restructured moment of its past" (Reader, 1997). In Mamdani's words, "Encased by custom, frozen into so many tribes, each under the fist of its own Native Authority, the subject population was, as it were, containerized" (Mamdani, 1996).

Reader means that everything that we call customary law—customary land rights, customary political structures and so on—was in fact invented through colonial codification. He expresses a utilitarian view of tradition: "Traditions in Africa and elsewhere are merely accepted modes of behaviour that currently function to the benefit of society as whole. They persist as long as their benefit is obvious, and fade away when it is not. Change and adaptability is the very essence of human life—nowhere more so than in Africa."

Indeed, things have changed. Mamdani describes the state that emerged through postindependence reform. Truly, it was not the same. However, "a version of a bifurcated state remained. For inasmuch as radical regimes shared with colonial powers the conviction to effect the revolution from above, they ended up in intensifying the administratively driven justice, customary or modern. Even when it was done in the name of development and waging revolution and there was a change in the name of the functionaries from chiefs to cadres, there was little change in the nature of power. The gulf between the town and country deepened."

In postindependence Tanzania, radical reform tended towards centralization. Initially thought of as voluntary political mobilization, this attempt to reform soon degenerated into a set of administrative decrees from above; such as when Tanzania proposed "the replacement of the matrilineal system of succession by a patrilineal one". Such attempts built on a colonial tradition of administrative justice and fused power. As the state bureaucracy prevailed over party officialdom, ideology and persuasion gave way to outright violence. The failed attempt at development from above degenerated into extra-economic coercion (Mamdani, 1996).

The political consensus centred on modernization and nationalism. The nationalist movement, and later the independent state, came to repress and undermine cultural and religious differences. Nyerere's modernizing theory rejected the past as traditional and inherited patterns of production as destructive and backward, despite evidence to the contrary. The common ground for consensus was limited to modernization. Yet the developmentalism of the nationalist movement became discredited because overt state regulation and control was basically inefficient and undynamic in character (Havnevik, 1993).

Since independence, the evolution of a national political identity has been stressed. In the name of national identity, the state discouraged rivalries on the basis of tribe, colour, and creed. The centralization process involved attempts to create a National Tanzanian Culture from culturally diverse communities. It also accentuated the use of Kiswahili as the national and official language over all other languages found in the regions and communities. Kiswahili is spoken and understood by most young people who have been to school. Among the older generation, this fluency is much less common. Tanzanian identity was emphasized above all local "ethnic" identities. While these efforts may have contributed to the development of a Tanzanian political identity, cultural differences between ethnic groups and regions remain.

The concept of tribe has been discredited as a colonial invention, an obstacle to modernization and/or as a threat to political unity. At present, many people avoid using the word tribe, preferring to use the name of their own ethnic group. "Ethnicity" has much of the same meaning as tribe, but avoids the pejorative implications of this term. It can be used to describe whole nations or small sub-tribes or communities (Peil, 1977). The concept of "identity" is also gaining ground.

Thus, tribes appear to be nonexistent and are centrally denied. However, community identities remain, especially in local cultural areas. Practices related to marriage and wedding rituals persist. Local languages and identities among such as the Sukuma, Haya, and others are very much alive. They shape perceptions and distinguish one Tanzanian from another. There are clear distinctions between rural and urban areas and between one urban area and another. The cultures of different communities are still breathing and vibrant. Customary practices on rights to land, the rights of women over inheritance of land, may conflict with the declared position of the Tanzanian state and its principles of gender equality and secularism. Tensions, therefore, remain and manifest themselves in marriages between individuals of different communities and religious persuasions over issues like bridewealth and individual choice of marriage partners versus arranged marriages. Tensions may become acute when one spouse dies.

It seems more likely that in future, as in the recent past, the solution to social problems has to draw on both traditional and contemporary resources. Tribes are not transhistorical. On the contrary, they are formed by their social-history, another name for tradition. Mamdani argues, that it would make sense to speak of the "making of an ethnicity". He underlines, that the rural-urban gulf can hardly be bridged by state enforcement, but by social processes that "transcend the unilinear modernist perspective that counterposes social particularism to state universalism". Our visits to rural communities tell of partial breakdowns of reproductive orders and the need to protect bonds between genders and generations.

Gender relations

The young girl in Tanzania has to contend with sexual harassment and sexual taboos. While customary instruction is impaired or absent, modern education has left the young in a vacuum. In "Teenage Mothers in their Second Pregnancies", Rosalia S. Katapa analyzes the circumstances and motives which lead to a second early pregnancy. She also looks at the young mother's chances of finding a good husband. The same crucial issue is also aired by the teenage boys interviewed by Juliana C. Mziray, the author of "Boys' Views on Sexuality, Girls, and Pregnancies".

Juliana Mziray talked to boys in a Kaguru and a Chagga village. The first village is predominantly matrilineal, with a poor and ill-educated population, the other patrilineal, with a comparatively well educated and well-off population. They are both growing business centres situated on thoroughfares. The boys discuss their perceptions of and experiences with girls since early puberty. Typically, they tell about a change in relations from companionship to rating girls as sexual objects and also to rating their moral standards. There is a striking contradiction between how boys conduct themselves and their prejudiced and condemnatory attitudes towards girls. The boys grow up under pressure to prove their manhood. Their peer-group not only accepts but demands sexual activity: having a girlfriend is regarded as a precondition of being seen as a man. Multiple partners and STDs are further proof.

When these attitudes are put into practice, the soil is prepared for gender antagonism. When the parents have lost their ability to influence the choice of husband or wife and the *deployment of alliances* is replaced by the *deployment of sexuality*, an unintended consequence is the evolution of a gender market for selection of partners (Holter, 1997). Young men and women meet, especially to begin with, in arenas like bars and discos. There they mix amidst of anonymous others. The crowd introduces an element of competition and ranking. Although the Norwegian sociologist Holter has studied partner choice in Norway, his observations seem valid of discos, bars, and similar meeting places in other societies, where marriages have become privatized and are no longer a concern of parents, kin, or clan.

The gender market is about partner selection. Here gender matters. The gendered choices are the most "strategic" choices of the whole gender system. The right balance of gender attraction and personal contact creates an institution for the individuals involved; it establishes a relationship among couples, perhaps even a family. Ultimately, young women and men go out to look for someone to love. Love, however, stands in contradiction to competition, the beauty game of rating and gaining attention as sexual objects and displaying "gendered attraction". Nevertheless, when individuals have identified each other they tend to develop more personal and exploratory relationships. Then it is time for them to withdraw from the "marketing game".

According to Holter, the rise of the gender market illuminates a seeming paradox in modern gender relations: increasing gender equality on the one hand, and an extension of money-for-sex transactions on the other. Prostitution and half-prostitution constitute a kind of backyard to the gender market. Whether increased gender-equality is valid outside Scandinavia, remains to be studied.

The interviews by Juliana Mziray describe how young boys enter the gender market and consume girls as objects of sexual desire, but end by being disappointed and begin considering the qualities desired in a wife. Yet they blame the girls for their frustration.

Considering the significance of partner selection, there is surprisingly little research on it. At least in the West, one suspects an attitude of avoidance, because the pleasant cultural images about partner selection tend to disregard the humiliations and risks of rejection inherent in marketing oneself.

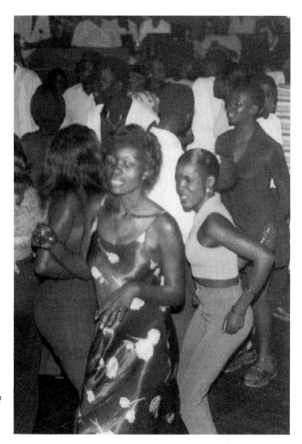

Young women and men mix amidst of anonymous others. The crowd introduces an element of competition and ranking.

(Photo Benny Kisanga)

Law and practice

In August 1985, Tanzania ratified the UN Convention on the Elimination of All Forms of Discrimination Against Women (CEDAW), which is a international human rights instrument on women's human rights. It has also been called the women's Bill of Rights. This UN treaty defines discrimination against women as meaning "any distinction, exclusion or restriction made on the basis of sex which has the effect or purposes of impairing or nullifying the recognition, enjoyment or exercise by women, irrespective of their marital status, on a basis of equality of men and women, of human rights and fundamental freedom in the political, economic, social, cultural, civil or any other fields" and requires state parties to take action to end discrimination against women in all sectors including abolishing discriminatory customary and religious laws.

However, studies have shown that people's attitudes and be-
haviours are still shaped from generation to generation by their customary patterns and by oral evidence. Indeed, the contribution by
Magdalena K. Rwebangira on "Maintenance and Care in Law and
Practice" indicates that people are still to a large extent influenced by
local customs and practices, despite the law to the contrary. This may
be due to ignorance of laws or lack of effective enforcement mechanisms of the modern laws, especially in remote rural areas away from
the modernization centres.

Urban poor

The present social context is one of increasing poverty and unemployment. These characterize many countries in the South, including
Tanzania. There is growing unemployment and retrenchment in
urban areas and a deterioration of rural conditions in the wake of
huge external debts and the decline in public education and public
health services.

In "Stone-breakers and Brick-lifters Aspiring for Earnings and
Families", Mary Ntukula illuminates the condition of rural girls who
have migrated to urban centres in search of menial jobs. She approached girls who have found a niche in the modern construction
sector. They occupy jobs which do not attract men, as the pay is low
and the work tedious. Yet these jobs give the girls some advantages
compared to domestic work. The author describes their daily realities,
health hazards, and dreams about earnings, marriage, and raising
families.

Petty activities, petty trading, prostitution, crime, and other illegal
activities have been high-lighted as some of the survival mechanisms
employed by those who tend to be marginalized and socially ex-
cluded. Despite the tension, the picture is not completely bleak.
People are not only affected by structures, but also act to influence
their conditions. The title "Relationships for survival" should be taken
literally. There is a common thread in the study on "Young Mothers
and Street Youth" by Virginia Bamurange: the need to have access to
significant others, e.g. people who one can trust and who take notice.
Even limited empathy and protection, and a reliable exchange make
sense compared to total neglect and indifference. Virginia
Bamurange's observations of interaction between mother and child,
and between street boys looking for human anchorage in an

anonymous and hostile urban environment, bears witness to something well known in principle yet frequently disregarded in practice.

Unsafe sexual relations

As societies in Africa change and adopt more and more of Western culture, teenage conduct has become unpredictable and problems which were rare before are more and more common. Teenagers are more free than ever to engage in sexual affairs. This puts them at risk of sexually transmitted diseases (STDs, including HIV/AIDS). Teenage morbidity and mortality has increased, with all the negative implications that entails. Young women who contract an STD may jeopardize their chances of bearing children. When these women get married, infertility may cause marital disharmony and divorce. Given the prevalence of the deadly HIV infection, it is alarming that more than 50 per cent of youth have had sexual intercourse by the age of 16. A recent study of university students, who are no longer teens, showed that although 90 per cent of them were having casual sex, very few used condoms and even fewer used condoms consistently. If university students who are considered adults and who are very aware of the risks from casual sex do not care, one wonders about teenagers who are expected to abstain from sex.

The economic crisis and attendant rising inflation hits adolescents hard. They may easily fall prey to material gifts aimed at luring them to engage in sex and will end up in trouble. Available information from private clinics shows that young girls with STDs are mostly infected by older men, sometimes old enough to be their grandfathers. Data collection on this issue is unsystematic except when problems occur. The teenager will not admit to having sexual relations with such men. Fear of parental disapproval inhibits the girls from disclosing information. This means that they report for treatment late, when the infection has already caused damage or, in the case of pregnancy, they resort to an unsafe abortion. Available data on female deaths indicate that 60 per cent of teenagers dying from abortion did so at home or arrived in hospital too late, because they tried to conceal the act. The ones who die are only the tip of the iceberg. For each one who dies there are probably ten who will have morbidity severe enough to leave permanent damage.

Problems of teenage pregnancy are not confined to the unmarried girls. Complications are known to be more severe in young teenagers, irrespective of their marital status. The girls are not ready physically and psychologically for pregnancy. Their growth is not yet complete. Problems such as severe hypertension and obstructed labour are common in pregnant teenagers. Table 1 shows that 21 per cent of women dying of pregnancy-related conditions were teenagers.

Table 1. *Distribution of maternal deaths by age and residence in urban and rural setting (%)*

Setting	Age of death				Number of cases
	–19	20–29	30–39	40–44	
Urban	15	46	39	0	13
Sub-urban	21	56	21	2	86
Rural	29	41	24	6	17
Missing	0	1	0	0	1
Total (%)	25 (21)	62 (53)	27 (23)	3(3)	117 (100)

From Urassa et al., 1995, *African Journal of Health Sciences*, 2:242–9

This age-group should be the target for education and counselling on matters related to sex. The current introduction of family life education may help in part. In some parts of the country, e.g., Zanzibar, parents consent to their teenagers getting married before finishing school. The implication is that these girls become mothers very young and experience complicated deliveries. The psychological trauma caused in some of these young mothers is immeasurable.

Pregnancy-related health problems are compounded by the fact that public opinion does not accept that adolescents have a premarital sex life. Young girls are supposed to abstain or to get married soon after menarche. Despite the fact that Tanzania officially allows the use of contraception by all sexually active individuals, young teenagers have little access to contraceptives. The teenager is often frowned upon if seen in a family planning clinic, especially if she is single. The consequence of this is unsafe abortion and death. Abortion is known to cause up to 24 per cent of the pregnancy-related deaths and together with haemorrhage, sepsis, and anaemia—all of which may occur due to the young age of mothers—constitutes more than half of the deaths among teenagers.

The reproductive health of male teenagers is rarely a topic of discussion. Young boys, curious about life, often experiment with sex. In town, prostitutes may be the first sexual contact. This encounter may lead to an infection. In other cases, boys experiment with teenage girls and the resulting pregnancy is often due to ignorance. Unfortunately for girls, it leads to the end of schooling. There is an increasing willingness today among politicians and parents to let girls continue with education after delivery. The growing movement of teenage boys from rural to urban areas also leads to boys having unprotected sex, with all its risks.

Table 2. *Cause of maternal death among women of reproductive age (%)*

| | Age | | |
	12–19	20–34	35–
Abortion	24	12	13
Haemorrhage	8	16	13
Anaemia	20	6	20
Sepsis	4	10	7
Hypertension	12	14	0
Other	32	42	47

From Urassa et al., 1996, *South African Medical Journal*, 96:436–44

Another important issue is the sexual abuse of teenagers. It is believed that both girls and boys are subject to sexual abuse. It is, however, young girls who are brought to hospital after they have been raped. Girls are raped by much older men and genital lacerations are common. It is estimated that at least five rape cases are reported daily to hospitals in Dar es Salaam alone. Many victims do not report and the incident goes unrecorded. The hazards of sexual abuse of teenagers may be great. Forced sexual intercourse may be painful. If it is the first contact, the teenager may associate sex with pain rather than pleasure. The psychological trauma resulting from rape may have far-reaching implications. There are reports of sexually transmitted diseases, including HIV infections, following acts of rape. In fact, sexual abuse of adolescents, with resulting genital lacerations, is an efficient way of transmitting HIV. It is now routine to screen all raped women immediately after the rape and then three months later in order to determine if the perpetrator infected the victim. Unfortunately, there are no laws requiring suspected rapist to have their blood taken for examination. The presence of street girls who are easy prey for multiple sex partners or indeed for sexual abusers will compound the issue. Sexual abuse may also lead to pregnancy. Among street teenagers, where abuse is not reported to hospitals, pregnancy often goes unnoticed until labour, too late for any intervention. In these cases, complications like anaemia are not noticed and the growing abdomen is attributed to overeating. The first sign of pregnancy may be facial swelling due to severe high blood pressure. Unwanted and unplanned pregnancies among street teenagers are more likely to result in problems, because the teenagers are uncared for and the usual social support available to ordinary women is lacking.

In some parts of Tanzania, girls are subjected to varying degrees of circumcision. Parts of the girls external sex organs are excised, usually without anaesthesia. Besides the pain, depending on the extent of excision there may be scarring and complications during future pregnancies. While tribes, such as the Wagogo, who still circumcise, defend the practice it in terms of womens' dignity, several national and international pressure groups are campaigning for an end to "mutilation, abuse and torture".

Sexual partners

In our studies, we have collected evidence about difficulties that young people face and risks that they expose themselves to in becoming sexually active. Thus, we focus on problems and those youths that experience difficulties, the bad news. Table 3 gives the reader an overview that prevents generalizations on the basis of our limited local data. Our data aim to promote understanding of and insight into the concrete and diverse conditions of some teenagers.

The 1994 *Knowledge, Attitudes and Practices Survey* (KAP) asked men and women about their sexual partners within the last twelve months. They were asked about their spouses, regular sexual partners other than their spouses, and non-regular partners. They were asked how many people they had sex with and when the most recent sexual encounter took place. A regular partner is someone with whom the respondent has been having sexual relations for a year or more. Unmarried men and women were asked whether and how many regular sex partners they had. They were also asked whether they had had sexual intercourse with someone other than a regular partner within the prior twelve months, and how many people they had sex with, and when the most recent sexual encounter with a non-regular partner occurred.

Table 3. *Number of sexual partners*

Percent distribution of women and men by number of person of the opposite sex with whom they had intercourse in the last 12 months and mean number of persons with whom they had sexual intercourse, 1994

Age	Currently married						Who are not currently married					
	Number of partners including spouse						Number of partners					
	0	1	2–3	4+	Total	Mean	0	1	2–3	4+	Total	Mean
Women												
15–19	6.4	88.1	5.4	0.0	100.0	1.0	76.6	18.5	3.3	1.6	100.0	0.3
20–24	5.2	86.1	7.6	1.0	100.0	1.1	61.8	32.7	3.6	1.9	100.0	0.6
26–29	5.0	87.3	6.9	0.9	100.0	1.1	47.0	39.2	12.0	1.9	100.0	0.9
30–39	6.7	86.5	5.7	1.1	100.0	1.1	56.9	33.1	7.2	2.7	100.0	1.0
40–49	8.2	87.2	4.6	0.0	100.0	1.0	68.6	27.6	3.8	0.0	100.0	0.4
Total	6.2	86.8	6.2	0.8	100.0	1.1	67.7	25.9	4.7	1.7	100.0	0.5
Men												
15–19	*	*	*	*	*	*	58.4	20.9	15.3	5.4	100.0	0.8
20–24	0.0	60.8	31.5	7.7	100.0	1.8	35.5	30.7	21.6	12.3	100.0	1.6
25–29	1.8	65.7	21.9	10.6	100.0	2.0	32.4	39.0	19.4	9.2	100.0	1.3
30–39	3.6	67.9	22.4	6.1	100.0	1.5	39.1	28.7	25.9	6.3	100.0	1.2
40–49	7.1	69.6	19.3	3.9	100.0	1.4	66.5	25.2	2.8	5.5	100.0	0.6
50–59	6.4	78.6	11.7	3.3	100.0	1.2	66.5	18.4	15.0	0.0	100.0	0.6
Total	6.4	78.6	11.7	3.3	100.0	1.5	66.5	18.4	15.0	0.0	100.0	0.6

Note: Married respondents who were not sexually active in the last 12 months are assumed to have been sexually active with their spouses

* less than 25 cases

Source: *Bureau of Statistics*, 1995. KAP Survey, Table 7.1 and 7.1.2

The vast majority of married women (93 per cent) had not had sex with anyone other than their spouse (or had not had sex at all) in the twelve months preceding the survey. Women who have had a partner other than their spouse fell into all age categories, educational levels, and had been married for widely different periods. Most of the un-married women who were sexually active in those twelve months had only one partner (26 per cent of all unmarried women). Unmarried women who had more than one partner are of all ages and educa-tional levels. Unmarried women aged 25–29 are most likely to have had more than one partner (14 per cent).

Men, both married and unmarried, are more likely than women to have had more than one sexual partner in the twelve months preced-ing the survey. About one-quarter of married men have had two or more partners; one-half of unmarried men had been sexually active in those twelve months; one-quarter of unmarried men had one partner, and one-quarter had two or more partners. The unmarried women and men who have had more than one partner in the previous twelve months are of all ages and educational levels. The likelihood of having two or more partners increases with increased education.

Social history and identity

Youth in Tanzania grow up in widely divergent social conditions. The split between urban and rural life affects the way they understand themselves and the content and traits from which they construct their identities. Modern youth identity predisposes the younger generation to freer and more unrestrained behaviour regarding love, coupling, and sex, as cultures and ways of life are transformed and incorporate new values.

New values of self-excellence and increased choice place teenagers in the unenviable position of having to cope with demands of new and old values, which may differ or be incompatible in regard to choice of marriage partner, relations with parents and kin, future careers and work away from home and birthplace. Under such cir-cumstances, the creative capacity of teenagers is constantly called upon.

What then, do we mean by "modern identity"? According to Giddens (1991), identity is based on a history of the self:

> Identity is not distinctive traits or features possessed by the individual. Identity is not something given but something that has to be routinely

created and sustained. A person with a reasonably stable sense of self-identity has a feeling of biographical continuity which she is able to grasp and to communicate to other people. It means that the individual's identity rests on her capacity to tell who she is, i.e., *to keep a particular narrative going*. As has been said: "In order to have a sense of who we are, we need to have a notion of how we have become, and of where we are going" [Giddens, citing Taylor, 1989]. Thus, self-identity presumes a narrative, a history about the self (pp. 52–4). The modern individual is the master of her identity, the one who creates herself by continuous self-observation and reflexion. We are not what we are, but what we make of ourselves (p. 75).

It is tempting to relate these claims about self-reliance and master-hood to observations about identity in the context of the evolution of modernity in European societies between 1750 and 1900. According to Bauman, (1993) another notable current sociologist:

Modern society did not differentiate and assign in the first place explicit identities, but rather varying measures of freedom of movement between identities, or ... *freedom to choose between identities*. However, that freedom was unevenly distributed. A relatively small proportion of the population came close to the choosers, rule-setters, the self-makers, the "individuals" in the strict sense of the word. The rest were not trusted with choice making, denied the ability to put freedom to an acceptable use. The great majority were "classified out" of moral self-management. "The rest", those without freedom to choose included inferior races, i.e., backward and childlike, the poor and indigent, i.e., moved by dark impulses rather than reason, women i.e., endowed with greater animality and less reason than their male counterparts (p. 120).

Encroachment took place in the colonies where traditional societies were ruled by customary law, as defined by the Native Authorities. Today, development ideology holds out the prospect of free choice, but in reality the choices are limited and conditional. Modern identity rests on certain rights and assets.

Let us look at a girl who is born in a rural area and grows up in a typical or semi-typical customary family, with its set of instructions to develop articulated values which are acceptable in the community. At a certain age, modernization exerts pressure on her and her family. She must join a formal system of education to learn how to read, write, and do arithmetic. There are social and economic expectations which go with these skills. She has both traditional and modern aspirations, just as her parents and the community have theirs of her. The church, another form of modernity, has its own form of education to

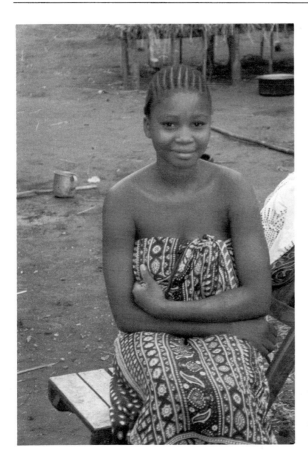

Young girls are to a
large extent objects for
other peoples choices.
(Photo Rita Liljeström)

promote its own set of values. It discards certain forms of customary knowledge and rural values and casts them as abstract "devils" to be fought.

In our fieldwork, we had a strong impression of a bifurcated state, where rural people are paying a heavy toll for past modernization. When politicians, political scientists, and economists analyze change, they tend to neglect the long-term impact of the erosion of previous moral orders and the loosening of mutual human bonds which protect minors, women, children, and aged people. We have reported on single mothers, maternal grandparents taking care of their daughter's out-of-wedlock children, on generational alienation, on young men refusing to marry yet repeatedly conceiving children whom they abandon, on STDs as proof of manhood, on marriages ending in divorce, and on girls generating money by sexual services.

The knowledge the rural girl acquires from her environment; the values she develops within her family and community; the information she garners from her religious experience, from her peer-group, from the mass media, and from her own experience, remain conflicting sources for self-making. Young girls are to a large extent objects of other people's choices. Where they are no longer part of the clan, they often engage in sexual relationships with men who avoid lasting commitments and they risk becoming pregnant out-of-wedlock. Alice K. Rugumyaheto has visited training institutions for unmarried teenage mothers and looked into their programmes and assets. She reports her impressions of the opportunities that are being opened to these girls in "Pregnancy is Not the End of Education".

Giddens gives expression to a common belief that in cultures where social conditions stayed more or less the same from generation to generation, change to social identity was clearly staked out, e.g., such as when an individual moved from adolescence to adulthood. Tradition and the small community provided a protective framework. It appears that hardly any individual notions existed. How far do collectively shared models leave room for a sense of individual freedom? How much scope did clan rule leave for its members to express and mould individual identities? These are questions posed by cultural anthropologist who study personhood and agency in African cultures.

Personhood in African cultures

In African tradition, it makes sense to distinguish between an official view of personhood, on the one hand, and the emotional experience of selfhood on the other (Jacobson-Widding, 1990). The official view embraces the moral person, i.e., personhood in terms of roles and rules, while the experience of selfhood rests on self-awareness. Here, personhood is treated as synonymous with "identity".

Anthropologists argue that in any society the ideologically supported idea of personhood entails a shadowy, unofficial, countervailing set of ideas and experiences. The counter-normative domain stands for comparative freedom. Whereas the official view of personhood may be presented publicly, the emotional experiences of personhood are expressed in ambiguous metaphors. For example, the metaphor of shadow among the peoples of Lower Congo is a perfect symbol of individual identity *when it is felt to be elusive*. In any village "people tacitly accepted rules of avoidance, in order to convey the message: 'Don't step on this image of myself', or: 'I am not going to offend you by stepping on your shadow'" (Jacobson-Widding, 1990: 31).

> When people explain why they try to avoid having other people step on their shadow, it seems that the fear of being stepped on is a fear of having one's own capacity of agency being caught or blocked by somebody else. The term used for such "blocking" is *bindika*, which means "to close" or "to bind". People tend to protect symbols of individuality in order to preserve their sense of vitality and agency.

> Besides the metaphors of shadow, there are other institutional devices which allow for expression of individuality and freedom, for instance the recognized metaphors like shape-shifting (i.e., individuals able to transform themselves into animals), states of spirit possession, and dance, to mention a few. Dance creates links between the vital energy of the individual body, the social body, and the cosmos. The sense of oneness which people get through dancing together follows from the way in which personal, social and cosmological meaning are brought into an all-encompassing communion (Jackson and Karp, 1990:22).

A conclusion that the anthropologists draw is that of the two complementary views of personhood, one may be defined as a sociocentric view while the other may be defined a egocentric. The former concerns the social roles of a person, while the latter expresses the emotional and interactional experiences of selfhood. The two views of personhood coexist in the same culture although one of them may dominate at the expense of the other.

One can go on and argue that two coexisting but non-comparable worlds, the *sacred* and the *profane,* provide means for self-expression and the remaking of the moral. Durkheim found that in "primitive" societies these two worlds were mutually isolated.

> He reflected over the smooth, peaceful and regular alterations of the *profane* and the *sacred,* of mundane everyday and carnival, structure and counterstructure. The separation made wonders: the profane, languishing and dull rhythm of everyday could replenish its energy, rejuvenate itself by year, swilling the water of life from the fount of popular emotions without being threatened in the intervals by the uncontrolled eruption of the crowd's frenzy. This peaceful and profitable cohabitation "puts clearly in evidence the bond uniting them to one another, but among the people called civilized, the relative continuity of the two blurs their relations"(Bauman, 1993:134).

> Durkheim looked desperately for the sources of moral vigour in his own European world of strict division of labour and professional separation.

He strongly believed that "moral remaking cannot be achieved except by means of reunions, assemblies, and meetings where the individuals, being closely united to one another, reaffirm in common their common sentiments" (Bauman, 1993:134).

While the anthropologist, Jacobson-Widding, explains a person's sense of vitality, creativity, and agency by her or his expression of autonomous selfhood in metaphors and celebrations, Durkheim identifies the moralizing and revitalizing power of shared sacred oneness. Both of them point to emotional experiences beyond the everyday and regard these elements as complementary and not as mutually exclusive.

How to reconcile custom and modernity?

What Durkheim feared in modern society was the ruthless assault of the profane against the sacred, reason against passion, norms against spontaneity, and structure against counter-structure. The new state-managed order saw all vestiges of local authority as disruptive. Cultural crusades of early modernity in Europe were aimed at uprooting and destroying the plural, manifold, communally sustained ways, in the name of one, uniform, civilized, enlightened, law-sustained pattern of life. What the crusades set out to extirpate was criticized as the "old" and "backward" modes of existence.

The war against the local, the irregular and the spontaneous was merciless. Serious efforts were made to replace manifold local gettings together, with their much needed function of replenishing the reservoirs of sacred unity, with centrally planned and controlled celebrities and calendar of festivities. As a rule they became focal points, symbols, and the rituals of the new religion: that of nationalism (Bauman, 1993:135).

In reading Bauman on Durkheim, it is striking to recognize the same modernizing contradictions in African societies: the ruthless assault of the urban against the rural, state against communities, nation against tribes, the educated elite against common people, modernity against custom, profane against sacred, individual values against communal values.

Conflicting values leave the youth at a crossroads, bereft and alone. To them, and genuinely so, there seem to be no values, whether traditional, religious, or modern that directly address their predicament. Nevertheless, contradictions and ambiguities are part of human life. They existed in traditional communities as well, and individuals

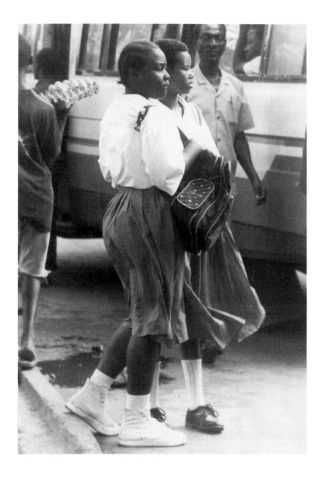

Urban schoolgirls
(Photo Benny Kisanga)

and collectivities had to invent methods to cope with them. Yet it appears as if the modernizing efforts abolish rituals and metaphoric beliefs that enable people to, if not solve, then at least to release tensions and cope with the ambiguities of existence.

In this study we have explored how teenagers understand themselves in relation to their passage from childhood to adolescence, and how they create their gendered self-image or identity by listening, observing, and trying to interpret the situations in which they find themselves. To get a glimpse of the social-history of the places where the teenagers live, we have added testimonies from people who were young very long ago. The emphasis has been on understanding what it means to be young in a rapidly eroding, resisting, and innovating social and cultural context.

Obviously, many sexual and reproductive health problems have their roots in deteriorating social relations. Part of the cure is restoring and recreating understanding and trust between genders and generations. Certainly there are ambiguities and contradictions even in the transformation of authoritarian relationships into responsive ones. Rosalia S. Katapa's suggestion about gender sensitization is worth considering. Although it is directed towards Nyakusa people, on the basis of her study, its validity is much broader. The modern concept "reflexivity", noted by Giddens, is another tool for overcoming the gulf between genders and generations, custom and modernity.

References

Amadiume, Ifi, 1997, *Reinventing Africa*. London: Zed.

Bauman, Zygmunt, 1993, *Postmodern Ethics*. Oxford: Blackwell.

Booth, D., et al., 1993, *Social, Cultural and Economic Change in Contemporary Tanzania*. Report to Sida commissioned through the University of Dar es Salaam and Stockholm University.

Brandström, Pär, 1990, "Seed and Oil: The Quest for Life and the Domestication of Fertility in Sukuma-Nyamwezi Thought and Reality" in Anita Jacobson-Widding and Walter van Beek (eds.), *The Creative Communion. African Folk Models of Fertility and the Regeneration of Life*. Uppsala: Uppsala Studies of Cultural Anthropology.

Foucault, Michel, 1978, *The History of Sexuality*. New York & London: Penguin.

Giddens, Anthony, 1991, *Modernity and Self-Identity*. Cambridge & Oxford: Polity Press.

Havnevik, Kjell J., 1993, *Tanzania: The Limits of Development from Above*. Uppsala: Scandinavian Institute of African Studies in cooperation with Mkuki na Nyota Publishers, Dar es Salaam.

Holter, Oystein Gullvåg, 1997, "Gender, Patriarchy and Capitalism". Unpublished Ph.D. thesis, University of Oslo.

Jackson, Michael and Ivan Karp, 1990, "The Experience of Self in African Cultures", in M. Jackson and I. Karp, *Personhood and Agency*. Uppsala: Uppsala Studies in Cultural Anthropology.

Jacobson-Widding, Anita, 1990, "The Shadow as an Expression of Individuality in Congolese Conceptions of Personhood", in M. Jackson and I. Karp, *Personhood and Agency*. Uppsala: Uppsala Studies of Cultural Anthropology.

Kaijage, F. and A. Tibaijuka, 1996, *Poverty and Social Exclusion in Tanzania*. Geneva: ILO.

Mamdani, Mahmood , 1996, Citizen and Subject, Contemporary Africa and the Legacy of Late Colonialism. Princeton Studies in Culture/Power/History. Kampala: Fountain Publishers.

Mbiti, John, 1969, African Religions and Philosophy. London: Heinemann.

Peil, Margaret, 1977, Consensus and Conflict in African Societies. London: Longman.

Reader, John, 1997, Africa, A Biography of the Continent. London: Hamish Hamilton.

Tanzania Demographic and Health Survey 1991/1992. Dar es Salaam: Bureau of Statistics.

Tanzania Knowledge, Attitudes and Practices Survey, 1994. Dar es Salaam: Bureau of Statistics.

Urassa, Ernest J.N., et al., 1995, African Journal of Health Sciences, 2:242–9.

—1996, South African Medical Journal, 96:436–44.

Chapter 2
Nyakusa Teenage Sexuality—Past and Present

Rosalia S. Katapa

Sexuality for procreation in most sub-Saharan countries starts during
the teenage years (Bledsoe and Cohen, 1993). These authors say that
"the most significant change in sub-Saharan Africa is not a rise in
overall rates of adolescent fertility but in childbearing among women
who do not appear to be married." This means that there has been a
shift in sexuality-for-procreation among adolescents from being
within marriage to being out-of-wedlock.

The focus of my research is Nyakusa teenage sexuality in the past
and at present. I identify conditions of teenage sexuality which are
continuing as well as those which have died out. The difference
between my research and other studies on the Nyakusa is that the
majority of our key informants were the present and former teenage
girls. Most research on Nyakusa has focused on either the society or
on men and key informants were mainly men. The studies were done
by outsiders with little or no knowledge of Kinyakusa (the Nyakusa
language), who depended on interpreters to a certain extent. I am
Nyakusa thus there were no language problems.

Literature on the Nyakusa dates back to the nineteenth century,
when the German missionaries arrived in Bunyakusa (the land of the
Nyakusa). According to Charsley (1969), "Nyakusa of southern Tanzania are among the best known of African peoples in the literature of
social anthropology." When Wilson visited Bunyakusa in the mid-
1930s she found that Banyakusa (the Nyakusa people) were practising
wife and husband replacement, commonly known as wife and husband inheritance:

> Formerly a marriage was a contract between lineages rather than
> between individuals. A girl was betrothed before puberty to a man of her
> father's choice and should he die she was still regarded as married to his
> heir. Should she die, a sister replaced her. Ideally a marriage bond
> between lineages lasted for generations, each man who died being

replaced by a brother or son, each woman by a sister or brother's daughter (Wilson, 1959).

She also found that brides were examined for virginity. Moreover, according to her, Moravian missionaries were reluctant to perform church weddings unless they were certain of the conduct of the bride and bridegroom. They preferred that a customary marriage be blessed by a church elder who was not a marriage officer; customary marriage did not involve vows. This was done in order to avoid difficulties in granting legal divorce if the wife was later deserted. The Moravian church was and still is the prominent church of Bunyakusa.

In the mid-1950s, when Wilson returned to Bunyakusa, she recognized that many changes had occurred. She noted that wife and husband replacement was not as widely practised as before. Christianity had spread widely. Nyakusa Christian men married only one wife and were not inheriting wives. She observed that although girls were still being betrothed before puberty, they did not go to their husbands until that time, and that divorce was more common than it had been twenty years earlier. Despite these changes, brides were still examined for virginity. "The traditional examination of the bride by the mothers and the giving of a bull if she goes to her husband a virgin are maintained in the Christian community. The bull is usually killed as a feast to the mothers to say thank you for nourishing her" (Wilson, 1959).

It is about forty years since Wilson's last visit to Rungwe district. Since then, there have been further political, economic, and social changes in Tanzania. There have been improvements in communication and transportation between Bunyakusa and other Tanzanian areas. The economic status of Nyakusa woman has improved because roads have reached remote areas of Bunyakusa; a woman is able to conduct a business, obtain an income, and reduce or eliminate her dependency on her husband. Such businesses include transporting and selling bananas in Tukuyu, Mbeya, Chunya, and Tunduma towns. Another emerging business is the buying of secondhand clothes in Mbeya and selling them in rural areas. The existence of roads in remote areas has contributed to improvements in social services by way of health centres and schools. Because of improved transportation, people (especially youths) run away from villages in search of employment in towns. Employment of Nyakusa men in the mines of Central and South Africa ceased in the mid-1960s. All these changes have probably affected Nyakusa sexuality.

My research objectives were to study Nyakusa teenage sexuality and update the literature on Nyakusa. As we have seen, prior to independence in 1961, there had been intensive social research among the Nyakusa, but since then not much in-depth research has been done.

Five main themes, two towns, three age categories of women and men

Our group was basically doing ethnographic research. We grouped our questions into five main themes, as follows:

1. Questions arising from reading the Wilson literature

In wife inheritance, did a teenage wife have a say? Who in the clan was entitled to inherit her and what criteria were used to select him? If she refused to be inherited, what actions were taken? In wife replacement, did the teenager replacing the deceased sister or aunt have a say and was bridewealth paid for her? What was the rationale for wife and husband replacement?

2. Questions about teenage sexuality in the past

How were girls and boys treated in preparation for their roles as adults? Who were their instructors and role models? At what age were girls generally betrothed? What was the marital and age status of their fiancés? How much bridewealth was generally asked and how much of it had to be paid before marriage took place? Who was entitled to take part in examining the bride for virginity? If the examination revealed that the bride was not a virgin, what action was taken?

Where there other forms of accession to marriage? What did marriage mean to the bride, bridegroom, their clans and communities? What roles were associated with a wife's rank in a polygamous marriage? Were women allowed to divorce their husbands? Were there marriage markets for divorced women? What were the repercussions when a wife ran away from her husband? What did a woman do once her husband ran away from her? Was there rape in Bunyakusa? Could rape lead to marriage?

3. Questions about teenage boys' sexuality

At what age did boys commence residing in age-villages? What was the significance of the age-villages? It is said that while Nyakusa girls married young, the boys married very late. Did they indulge in sex before marriage?

4. Questions about taboos related to sexuality

Were there sex taboos in Nyakusa culture? How were those who broke them punished?

5. Questions about current teenage sexuality

Currently, how are girls and boys treated in preparation for their roles as adults? Is the Moravian church still reluctant to perform church weddings? Is the marriage age still puberty? What are the implications of formal education, improved roads, and mixed marriages (marriages in which one partner is not Nyakusa) on Nyakusa teenage sexuality?

To find answers to such questions, Nyakusa women and men were interviewed. They belonged to three age categories, i.e. old, middle-aged, and youths. The old respondents were above 55; this age being chosen as a cut-off point because it is the compulsory retirement age in Tanzania. The middle-aged respondent were between 30 and 55 years old and youths were between 15 and 29. Altogether, data were collected from eight old people (four women and four men), six middle-aged people (four women and two men), and ten youths (six women and four men). The justification for having more female than male respondents is that, in addition to providing general information on teenage sexuality, they narrated their marriage histories. Similarly, we talked to more youths than old and middle-aged people because we wanted to learn more about current teenage sexuality from them.

We used open-ended questions in the interviews. The old and middle-aged Nyakusa answered questions on past and current teenage sexuality, the youths dealt only with current teenage sexuality. The questions were in Kiswahili. Interviews were conducted in Kiswahili or Kinyakusa or a mixture of both languages, according to the wishes of each respondent. All my research assistants were Banyakusa. Despite the language options in the interviews, the questionnaires were completed in Kiswahili.

The study was conducted in Tukuyu and Mbeya towns, the reason being that they are at different stages of urbanization.

Different types of marriage

The upbringing of the girls was geared to making them good wives and mothers. Girls were taught domestic work, handicraft such as weaving mats, and they worked on farms alongside their mothers and looked after the youngsters. Most of the skills were imparted to a girl by her own mother in particular and by all "mothers" in the community. If a girl lived with her grandmother, the grandmother was the one who had the primary responsibility of imparting the skills to the granddaughter. Girls were encouraged to be hardworking and were warned that it was not easy for a lazy girl to get a good husband.

Engagement to an unborn child

In Bunyakusa, part-payment of the bridewealth effected engagement; the initial deposit was at least one cow. At the time when the old men and women were growing up, it was possible to become engaged to an unborn child: a man predicting that a pregnancy would result in a girl child, would pay the initial deposit. Once, an engagement happened in this way it was usually about twelve years before the marriage took place. A man aged 57 declared that he had engaged an unborn child and later married her. It was common for girls under twelve years to be engaged. Most of the old and middle-aged people said it was rare for a girl to refuse to marry the man her clan had selected. When that happened, she was beaten until she accepted the marriage, failing which she was chased away from her father's home and the bridewealth was refunded.

Ukwakumbika: formal marriage

At the time the old women and men were growing up, six to seven cows had to be paid as bridewealth in order for a marriage to take place. In addition, one bull had to be given in advance as a price to the girl's "mothers" (female neighbours and aunts) because she was a virgin; it would be returned if examination proved otherwise. Before the wedding, the bride was given presents by her clan and female neighbours. The presents included special oils (*inyemba isyunguti*) for softening her skin, mats (*indeefu*) for sleeping or lying on, and household items such as pots, winnowing baskets, and wooden serving spoons (*miko na upawa*). By then she would also have made some mats for herself.

The day before the wedding, the bride was admonished by her mothers. She was told that upon marriage she had to obey her husband, satisfy him sexually, not refuse anything he said, not reply to him when he was angry, love his clan, and to keep the house and compound clean. She was told how to take care of herself during pregnancy, what to expect during labour, and how to endure it. A 70-year-old Mbeya woman provided further information about admonition; she said it was a regular occurrence while she was growing up. Girls would regularly be gathered and taught the norms of life, i.e., good behaviour.

A Nyakusa bride was examined for virginity either the evening before or early on the morning of her wedding day. Her "mothers" conducted the examination, and her own mother was never a member of the examining team. According to Nyakusa custom, this first examination was not absolutely necessary. The bride was subjected to another examination after or during the wedding ceremony. This one was conducted by the bridegroom's "mothers". The second examination was confirmation by the bridegroom's clan that she was indeed a virgin and hence that her clan deserved the bull and the other gifts already given. The biggest reward the bride received for being a virgin was *akalulu*, i.e., ululation, Monica Wilson (1952) called this the "cry of triumph". The whole place rejoiced at the sound of the ululation. Other presents included money and clothes. On the other hand, if the examination revealed that the bride was not a virgin, there were no presents. If the bridegroom claimed that he had not deflowered the bride, a light sentence would be passed on her clan whereby they would return the bull to the bridegroom's clan.

In many cases, the bridegroom's clan refused the bride because accepting her meant bringing much shame on them. If a prospective non-virgin bride was to be the first wife, she would almost always be refused.

For the bride the wedding confirmed that she was now a wife and thus deserved the respect due to a wife by society. As for her clan, the wedding confirmed the good upbringing of the bride. For the bride's part, the wedding ceremony started at her parents' home where people assembled to eat and dance. Later people moved to the bridegroom's parents' home, taking the bride and her belongings with them. They carried food and local beer to be eaten and drunk by the bridegroom's people. For the bridegroom's part, people on his side assembled at his parents' home, prepared food and displayed it in a room where the local beer was stored. This food and beer would be exchanged for that brought by the bride's people. When the bride's party arrived, all joined together in dancing and exchanged the food and beer. The ceremony continued till late at night.

After marriage, the bride became responsible for all household chores, seed-planting, grass-weeding and crop-harvesting. During her spare time she would make mats.

The type of marriage I have been describing is called *ukwakumbika*. It is the formal, socially accepted type of marriage in Bunyakusa. For Christians, the only addition was that on the wedding day, instead of the bride's party going straight to the bridegroom's parents' home to meet his party, the meeting took place in the church. After the church proceedings were over, both parties went to the bridegroom's parents' home for the celebrations.

Ukunyaka: Marriage by grabbing or seizing

Some men decided to seize or grab their fiancées. The only reason given for this form of marriage was that many men could not afford the full bridewealth needed for a formal marriage. A delay in paying the required bridewealth would allow another man to marry her and lead to a refund of what bridewealth the first man had paid. Thus, poor men felt that the only option left for them was to snatch or seize their fiancées. Thus fiancée-seizure or snatching was associated with failure to pay all the required bridewealth and fear of losing the fiancée. A man would request his friends to keep surveillance of the movements of his fiancée. Once an opportunity arose, he would hide himself while his friends snatched her, whereupon he would emerge. They usually carried her shoulder high to his parents' home. As to how many men were involved in this snatching process, we were told that it depended on how well-built she was: usually it required three to five men.

After seizing her, she was taken to the "bridegroom's" parents who called together few female neighbours and a male go-between (*mshenga*). The go-between took a formal message to the "bride's" parents to inform them that she had been seized and was at her in-laws' home. The "bride's" parents called her "mothers" and their own male go-between and informed them of what had happened. The "mothers" and the "bride's" go-between went to the "bride's" in-laws. Upon arrival an examination for virginity was conducted. Once virginity had been confirmed, the "mothers" and the "bride's" go-between demanded to be given a certain amount of money to go back with, and made arrangements about when the bull should be paid, usually within a month. As for the rest of the bridewealth, it was agreed that it would be paid later. The term used for such an arrangement was *bikukabaga bosa,* which means that the bride and groom would together raise the bridewealth.

If fiancée seizing took place where the "bride" and "groom" were sexually acquainted, she was taken straight to the groom's house instead of his parents' home. Later the groom sent a message to his parents that he had seized his fiancée. They in turn sent a message to her parents. The "bride's" go-between went to the man's parents for negotiations about when the bull and other gifts should be paid. The "brides" "mothers" did not go to the "bridegroom's" parents' home, the reason being that there was no examination for virginity.

Sometimes beatings accompanied fiancée seizure. This was especially the case if a reluctant "bride" tried to free herself from the snatchers. At times, the beatings resulted in serious injuries. In other cases, a girl being snatched cooperated so willingly that her snatchers walked with her instead of carrying her shoulder high or dragging her. She might escape from her snatchers and run back to her parents. The outcome was that her father sent a message to the boy's father informing him that he wanted a formal marriage for his daughter. Some fathers also agreed to postpone their demands of more bridewealth. A few fathers threatened to break the engagement by refunding the bridewealth that had already been paid. The seizing of a fiancée as a form of marriage was not highly regarded. The reason being that it did not comply with the customary rules of marriage.

Christmas, new year, and other important occasions such as Queen Elizabeth's birthday used to be celebrated at the central public grounds in Tukuyu. The grounds used to be full of people. There were also local dances and feasting. These occasions provided the best conditions for seizing a fiancée. I first saw a girl being grabbed by a group of young men during one of those ceremonies. There followed a chorus of *bikunnyaka, bikunnyaka,* meaning they are grabbing or snatching her. That was in the late 1950s.

In villages far removed from Tukuyu town, fiancée-grabbing took place in the morning when the girl went to draw water from the well or late in the day when she was coming back from collecting firewood. When fiancée-grabbing took place, the girls with her could not get her back, because they did not have the strength of the men! Upon arrival home, they would break the news to her parents. Fiancée-seizing also took place at local dances such as *umpalano,* which was a dance for celebrating harvests.

Ukujonga: eloping

At times, when a boy and a girl were in love and the boy could not afford the bridewealth, they would elope. The girl may have sensed that most of the girls she grew up with were already married and she was not getting any proposals. Rather than remain unmarried, she opted for eloping once that option arose. After eloping, most couples went to the copper mines in Zambia (nkambofi) or gold mines in Chunya (kumbibwe) or tobacco farms in Tabora (kungambo).

When they realizing that their daughter had eloped, her parents started investigating who she had eloped with. Once they had gathered enough information on the boy, they approached his parents for bridewealth. His parents would make it clear that they had not been part of the deal. Then the groom's parents might pursue one of several courses of action:

- paying fines on the behalf of their sons;
- paying part of the bridewealth;
- asking to be given time to find their son, who would then save towards the bridewealth;
- declaring that they did not have any bridewealth to pay; or
- by reacting defiantly by saying "I do not have convincing evidence that my son has run away with your daughter."

In some cases, the girl's parents failed to uncover who had eloped with their daughter. They reported the matter to the judicial system (*baraza*) so that whenever the man was caught he would be taken to court. If he was not willing to pay bridewealth, he would be fined. This type of fine used to be two cows. In some cases, married women eloped too. The reasons for this will be discussed under runaway wives below.

Ukukoligwa na kingoli: rape

The four old and three middle-aged respondents confirmed that rapes had occurred in Bunyakusa. In Kinyakusa, a rapist was called *kingoli*. What actions were taken against a rapists? Once caught, a rapist was initially beaten by the community as a serious warning that what he had done was wrong. He was forced to marry the girl, the reason being that she was no longer a virgin. Who would marry her now that she had no "value"? In cases where a rapist refused to marry the victim and could not pay the fine, he was imprisoned. An additional non-material punishment was seclusion and being ridiculed by the community.

When a man raped a small child, he was beaten, taken to court, remanded, and later imprisoned. If the final punishment was not imprisonment, villagers felt that the legal system had "failed"; they chased him out of their village and barred him from returning.

If a girl had been raped by a stranger, there was a manhunt. Once found, the man was beaten and taken to court. Otherwise, people reported the case to the judicial system so that if the man was later caught, he would be taken to court. A place where rapists (usually strangers) commonly lay in wait was the forest where girls collected firewood. For this reason, girls were frequently warned to walk in groups. Girls were raped while going to draw water at wells or river banks and while walking near dark corners (*vichochoroni*). If a raped girl managed to get married later, she fetched less bridewealth because her value had declined due to her loss of virginity.

After a rape, the girl was massaged (*walimkanda*) with hot water and certain leaves. This was done to hasten the healing process. Sometimes, she was given local herbs in addition to the massage. The girl was also consoled by her family.

In some instances, rape resulted in marriage: as a wife, the victim had to follow all the Nyakusa customs of obeying and respecting her husband! I am aware of two Nyakusa rape cases which ended in marriage. One of them happened in the late 1960s in Tukuyu town and the other one in mid-1980s in Dar es Salaam.

Marital dissolution

Divorce

Divorce used to occur among the Banyakusa. Usually, it was accompanied by the return of part or all of the bridewealth. It was common for a divorced woman to be married again, but marrying a man who had never had a wife was unheard of. When divorce occurred, three things determined how much bridewealth would be returned. These were the number of children the woman had given birth to, the duration of the marriage, and the reasons for the divorce.

Husband/wife desertion

Elopement resulted in a deserted spouse. Some married persons deserted their spouses for reasons other than elopement. A wife who ran away from her husband either went to her parents or to a distant land on her own: she was running away for reasons other than having found another man. Each of the four old and three middle-aged women mentioned the husband's cruelty, including wife beating, as the main reason behind desertion. The other reasons mentioned were:

- the laziness of the husband, which caused hunger in the household;
- not being able to conceive;
- husband not providing for the material needs of his wife;
- the husband having concubines;
- the wife being given a lot of hard work, usually farmwork; or
- the husband being a drunkard or a thief.

The deserted husband faced great shame once it was known that he had been abandoned by his wife. His first step used to be to establish the whereabouts of his wife. If she had run to her parents, he would go there and explain what had gone wrong. Her parents and some elders would try to reconcile them. If there had been serious issues which had made her run away, the husband was fined a cow. Once the fine was paid, the wife would be escorted to her husband. She would bring food and local beer for her husband and his neighbours. Alternatively, if the wife's clan felt that her life would be in danger if she returned, the man was told to go to court. In court, the wife's father would admit that his daughter had come back to him. The court would then determine the amount of bridewealth to be refunded. If the court established that the husband's behaviour was terrible, it would order that his in-laws not refund him anything. It would also rule that once his ex-wife remarried, the bridewealth would go to her ex-husband to refund him his bridewealth.

The middle-aged women replied that the parents of a runaway wife, if they realized that she had been at fault, would not wait for the husband to come for her but would force her to go back to him. If the wife run away to an unknown destination, the husband went to court for a search warrant.

As for wife desertion, husbands sometimes ran away from their homes when they felt that they could no longer maintain their families. Another cause of wife desertion was when a husband went to a distant land in search of work and stopped communicating with his family. The wife would go to court to claim that she had been deserted. The court would usually tell her to wait for a specific period (usually two years). If he had not returned or communicated by that time, the court declared her divorced. It was her choice whether to remain unmarried or to look for someone else to marry.

Death of a husband and wife inheritance

Once a husband died, his wife was inherited by one of his brothers. She could not refuse because this practice was part of Nyakusa culture. The decision about who should inherit her was made at a special clan meeting. Preference was given to the brother immediately following the deceased man in birth order. If the deceased man did not have a full brother, a half-brother inherited her provided he was of good character. If he was not, cousins were considered. These were paternal cousins. Some respondents said the only eligible maternal cousins were those born of the deceased man's aunts. The reason behind wife inheritance was to bring the children up together with the late husband's brother's children to continue the relationship between the two clans, and not to forego the bridewealth.

When the old women and men were growing up, it was impossible for a widowed woman to refuse to be inherited, except if she was a teenager without children. On the other hand, when the middle-aged Nyakusa were growing up, refusal did occur, although very rarely.

Death of a wife and husband inheritance

If a wife died, her clan replaced her by giving her husband another wife (husband inheritance). The bride was either her younger sister or her niece (brother's daughter). This woman could not refuse the marriage. A young sister by a stepmother could be considered in the absence of an unmarried full sister. The main reason for husband inheritance was for the younger sister to take care of her late sister's children: in other words the children would feel that they had their "mother" around. When the old people were growing up, bridewealth was not paid for the new bride. As time went by, parents began charging a little bridewealth.

Adultery

Adultery was committed by Banyakusa. Once caught, the adulterous couple were beaten. Divorce or paying a fine to the husband or separation was the punishment meted out to an adulterous woman. Sometimes, separation led to divorce and at other times the woman was forgiven. Once forgiven, she was escorted to her husband by her "mothers" who carried food and local beer to be eaten and drunk by her husband and his neighbours.

An adulterous man paid cows as a fine (*ukuposola*) to the woman's husband. If the woman was unmarried, he was forced to marry her, or pay a fine in cows to her father. At times, he also paid local beer to the elders as a fine for misbehaving.

Teenage boys' sexuality

Kilumyana: Age-villages

After reaching the age of about 10, boys moved to their own huts in a special area. Since most of the boys living in that area were about the same age, this area was called *kilumyama*. The Wilsons (1957, 1959, 1970) translated this as "age-village". A better translation is "boys' age-village". Living on their own was the beginning of independence for the boys and a sign of their growing up.

Some people, including researchers, have asked "how is it that Nyakusa girls married young while the boys married very late?" Obviously, girls married young because their fathers wanted to get cows (bridewealth) as early as possible. My research confirms that boys married late because they could not afford the bridewealth of six to eight cows and a bull. Many Nyakusa boys had to earn money with which to buy cows for bridewealth. They went to different places looking for the jobs which would eventually fetch them wives. Within Tanzania, they went to gold mines in Chunya (*kumbibwe*), tobacco farms in Urambo (*kungambo*) as well as tea estates within the Rungwe district. Some boys went to the copper mines in Zambia (*nkambofi*) and others to gold mines in South Africa (*kujoni*). Whenever the Banyakusa said *kujoni* they meant Johannesburg. Realizing that many Nyakusa young men were seeking employment, a recruiting centre for South African mines (*Wenela*) was opened in Tukuyu. It closed after independence because the new government banned all forms of association with apartheid South Africa.

Nyakusa girls married young and most of them married old men because they were the ones who could afford the bridewealth. Over the years, the old men had accumulated cows from bridewealth for their daughters and, to a certain extent, through the sale of farm products. The following song tells of the fate of a young man who had fallen in love with a girl called Nyondo.

Song 1   *Nungwe Nyondo gwe, abakangali bakwege* (twice)
              Linga nali kujoni, pongali ngukwega (twice)

In this song the lover tells his girlfriend Nyondo that he is unable to marry her, and she should marry an old man: had he been in Johannesburg working in the mines, he would be able to marry her.

This song was created at a time when young men were poor and they could not afford wives because bridewealth was so high. On the other hand, old men were "rich", they had accumulated wealth. The only rich young men were the ones who had just come back from the mines in Johannesburg.

Despite the fact that Nyakusa boys married very late, they made love to women much earlier than that. Three categories of women have been identified by the old and middle-aged interviewees as having been the "women friends" of young unmarried men. They were the prostitutes, divorcees, and widows. Some men flirted with their fathers' junior wives. Prostitution was not rampant in Bunyakusa, but a few divorced women moved to towns and became prostitutes. As the following two songs show, prostitutes were despised:

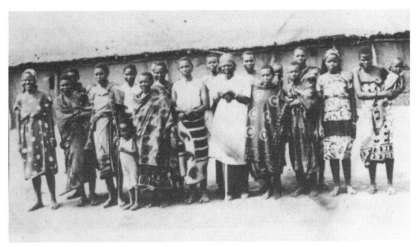

An African chief with all his wives.   (Photo *Daily News*, Dar es Salaam)
The old men marrying many wives post-
poned the marriages of the young men.

Song 2   *Gwabomba, gwabomba, Monica* (twice)
                Kumapipa, kumapipa Monica (three times)
                Gwakyaja, Gwakyaja, Monica (twice)
                Kumapipa, kumapipa, Monica (three times)

Translation   You have worked, you have worked, Monica
                At the drums, at the drums, Monica
                You have worked, you have worked, Monica
                At the drums, at the drums, Monica

This song was sung as a warning to girls not to get involved in prostitution. It tells of a girl called Monica who loitered as a prostitute. It
used to be said that hooligans and loiterers slept in *mapipa*, i.e., in
huge iron drums usually used for storing oil or tarmac. *Kumapipa*
meant a secluded place for storing empty drums where hooligans and
loiterers found refuge at nights.

Song 3   *Konala jope, Aliko Konala kuMbeje*

Translation   Konala, that one, there was Konala in Mbeya

The above line used to be sung as often as possible. Konala was the
first Nyakusa woman to practise prostitution. She found that it was

impossible to do so in Bunyakusa because it was contrary to local culture. She ran off to Mbeya where she became a prostitute.

To a slight extent, some men, single or married, surprised women
and raped them. Such behaviour by young men and their set was
against Nyakusa norms. Once found out, these men were punished.
Some old people in Mbeya maintained that although Nyakusa boys
married late, many of them did not indulge in sexual intercourse. The
reason for this is that they matured late, they were full of lice (*bali
bakololofu*), and they feared being reprimanded by their fathers.

When a Nyakusa young man had managed to raise enough cows
for bridewealth, the girl he was to marry was identified. Bridewealth
was paid to her clan and a wedding was arranged. The day before the
wedding took place, he was admonished by his "fathers", i.e., male
neighbours and uncles. During the admonition, he was told to love
his wife, not to be cruel to her, and to respect his marriage. He was
also told not to resort to beating his wife in cases of misunderstanding: instead he should call upon elders to effect a reconciliation.
He was advised to work hard so that he could take care of his wife, so
that she did not run away, and people did not despise him. The
bridegroom saw his wedding as confirmation that he was now an
adult (if this was his first marriage) and thus, deserving of the respect
due to a man. The wedding also confirmed that the bride had become
his property.

Polygamy

In the past, Nyakusa society was primarily polygamous. The first wife
had a special status and so did the youngest wife. The first wife had a
separate house in the compound and she was in charge of receiving
guests, including her husband's, and her own relatives. She allocated
the duties to the other wives, including preparing food for guests. She
kept the secrets of the household. Apart from her husband, she was
the only who knew where his spear was kept. Spears were the
weapons of war. One taboo was that she was not supposed to mix
with the other wives and they in turn were supposed to respect her.
Her house was the centre of ceremonies such as weddings and
mournings. Her first son was the successor to her husband's "throne".
The youngest wife, usually a teenager, accompanied her husband on
almost all his trips. Because of this, she was considered to be the
favourite wife.

Taboos related to sexuality

Women were not allowed to eat cockerels. A cockerel was equated with the father-in-law, and eating it was regarded as being disrespectful to him. It was believed that if a woman ate a cock, she would be cursed. In addition, the middle-aged respondents mentioned the following taboos:

- A wife was not supposed to walk behind her husband for fear of making him unsuccessful in all his endeavours:
- A wife had to avoid her father-in-law, otherwise she would give birth to weak and sickly children;
- A married woman should not only avoid seeing her father-in-law but also not mention his name. Upon his death, she had to avoidance to his grave, i.e., she was not supposed to see his grave;
- Once a girl got married, she was not allowed to use plates and utensils (*vyombo*) from her parents' home; she was considered to be dirty if she did so; and
- Finally, if a woman gave birth to twins, it was considered a bad omen and she was put into seclusion. After about two months, a local medicine man was called to perform a purifying ritual.

Current teenage sexuality

Girls are given an education which will lead to employment, formal or informal. This process will make them less dependent on their future husbands. Most girls find their own fiancés. Out-of-school girls start getting married at 15 years. On average, a girl's age at marriage is at least 18 years. Two young girls warned that it becomes difficult for a Nyakusa girl to be married after a certain age: one of them mentioned 25 to be the age and the other one believed it to be 29. Three cows are normally paid as bridewealth before a wedding takes place. In some instances, depending on the understanding between the two clans, two or only one cow can be paid.

Each of the five youths stated that brides are not now examined for virginity. The reasons advanced are that girls are "naughty", hence they are not virgins at the time of marriage. Three of the five youths added that "once engaged, they have sexual intercourse with their fiancée." Another said that "by not examining brides for virginity mothers avoid embarrassment." The Moravian church is opposed to examination of brides for virginity, and unlike in the past, encourages

church weddings. The reasons given for the church's change in attitude are that the majority of the Nyakusa are Christians and educated,
whereas before the majority were pagans and uneducated.

Ukwitwala: bringing herself

The old and middle-aged people identified a new form of marriage. It
is called *ukwitwala*. In an *ukwitwala* marriage, the plan involves only
one person, i.e., the bride. Even the man may not know that he is soon
be a "bridegroom". What normally happens is that there is friendship
between a man and the girl. Either due to false promises of marriage
or after becoming pregnant, the woman decides to leave her home
and go to the man's home. Initially, the man will think that he is being
visited by his girlfriend, especially if she decides to come empty-
handed or with only her handbag. As night approaches, he may even
tell her that it is getting late. She may reply "it is allright", and she
ends up sleeping there. The following morning, if requested to leave
she refuses, claiming that she will be chased away by her parents or
brothers for having slept out. Eventually, she becomes a wife and he
slowly pays bridewealth. Some of the middle-aged women and young
girls had this type of marriage. On a cautionary note, some of the girls
who attempt marry via the *ukwitwala* route are unsuccessful and are
left frustrated.

Mixed marriages

A non-Nyakusa man follows Nyakusa customs of betrothal if a
Nyakusa girl is involved, but the customs adopted after marriage, depend on where the couple live. If they live in Bunyakusa, they follow
Nyakusa culture to a great extent. Similarly, in mixed marriages
where the husband is Nyakusa, the couple are bound to follow the
culture of the place where they live. In most mixed marriages, there is
a tendency to follow the husband's culture more closely than the
wife's, no matter what place of residence. This means that Nyakusa
women married to non-Nyakusa men and not living in Bunyakusa are
at the greatest risk of losing their culture and traditions. One respondent said mixed marriages "pollute" Nyakusa culture, and that if they
become more common the Nyakusa culture may disappear.

Out-of-wedlock pregnancies

Out-of-wedlock pregnancies were rare in the past. The following reasons were given by the youths to account for their current prevalence:

- Girls are after money because of economic hardships;
- Poor upbringing of girls, unlike in the past;
- Education has contributed to changing the culture and traditions of the Nyakusa, to the extent that girls feel free to do whatever they want;
- Girls being given false promises by men who desert them after impregnation; and
- Girls having despaired of marriage because men are not proposing to them, finally deciding to have out-of-wedlock pregnancies so that they do not miss both marriage and children.

The old and middle-age people blamed education as a major cause of out-of-wedlock pregnancies.

Other issues

Rape and adultery still occur in Bunyakusa. Eloping and fiancée seizing rarely occur. All the youths said that wife inheritance had stopped while some old and middle-aged women claimed it was being practised on a very small scale. Husband inheritance does not exist any more. The reasons given for ending of the practice were:

- People are afraid of catching diseases, including AIDS;
- Change of culture and traditions, and law which leads to greater freedom for every person; and
- People are afraid of bearing more children because of the economic hardship in raising them.

The divorce rate is high compared to the past. Reasons contributing to this according to the youth are:

- Women's love of money, so that if the husband is poor, the Nyakusa woman will cause trouble until they divorce;
- Marriage infidelity;
- Educated women not being prepared to live in subordination to a husband;
- Wife-beating, rationalized on the basis that the husband paid bridewealth for the wife;

- Infertility in either partner; and
- Women's economic empowerment. Husbands feel that their wives are becoming assertive because of their financial power in the households.

The old and middle-aged respondents noted that many divorced couples had just been living together, i.e., bridewealth had not been paid for the wife, so the marriage bond was lacking. They also said that marriage is not as widely revered as it used to be and that tolerance is now lacking in marriage.

Types of marriage among the women interviewed

In the table below, the types of accession to marriage of the women we interviewed are presented. Information on the type of entry into marriage was not collected from the men.

Types of accession to marriage of the women respondents

Age group	Type of marriage Formal and socially accepted	Other types
Old	2	2
Middle-aged	1	3
Youths	1	5

Judging from the number of middle-aged and young women who were not married in formally accepted ways, it is clear that "lesser" forms of marriage are becoming common. It appears that, as time goes by, the socially accepted form of marriage is losing ground to lesser forms. Many girls are no longer waiting at home, while their fathers try to negotiate wedding plans for them. They make their own plans by eloping or moving in with their boy-friends. Others collude with their boyfriends to be seized.

Discussion

Institutions that regulate Nyakusa sexuality have changed over the years. I isolate a few issues from the research findings. According to Nyakusa culture, a boy's father and paternal uncles are responsible for paying bridewealth for his first wife. I will critically examine the reason given by the interviewed women and men that Nyakusa boys marry late because they could not afford bridewealth. Some people suggest that fathers and uncles did not provide bridewealth to the boys because they were themselves interested in the same girls. Indeed, it is the old men who married most of the girls. Other people said that bridewealth was the Nyakusa institution for delaying marriage for boys so there was a gap between the husband's and first wife's age. It was noted by some respondents in Mbeya town, that although Nyakusa boys married late, they did not indulge in sexual intercourse because they matured late and were full of lice. If fathers accepted that belief, then the theory of not providing bridewealth for boys as an institutional way of delaying marriage holds water.

Rape is viewed as a bad thing to happen to anyone and that is why the Nyakusa had stiff punishments for rapists. What is surprising is that the main punishment for the rapist was being forced to marry his victim! This must have been very humiliating for the poor woman. How could she respect and obey the rapist-turned-husband? This practice makes one realize that Nyakusa culture was very oppressive towards women. The practice of the rapist marrying his victim has not died out. The justification that the rapist has destroyed the girl's virginity and therefore must marry her is questionable. Rape can continue after marriage. Since rape in marriage is not fully acknowledged in many societies, the poor woman could continue to suffer without redress. In my opinion, the Nyakusa should concentrate on counselling the victim rather than think of the bridewealth her father would forego after the misfortune.

It appears that if adultery was committed, the woman's husband was viewed as the victim. The wife of a adulterous man was never viewed as a victim. This also underlines how Nyakusa culture favoured men.

The divorce rate has increased. Not all unmarried girls get a chance to marry, and the implication is that for divorced women the chances of remarrying are much lower. Thus there is suffering among divorced women due to economic hardship. It is known that Banyakusa women do not own land, and even if they go back to their parents they are not generally given land to till. The outcome is that many of them run away to towns or the city. Those who are lucky become barmaids, but some of them find themselves practising prostitution. My earlier research (Katapa, 1993) showed that divorced women are significantly overrepresented in urban areas in comparison to married ones. Other repercussions of divorce are on the welfare of children. Informal studies have shown that most of the street children in Tanzania are from broken homes. Indeed, many children find it intolerable to live with their divorced mothers who face severe economic hardship. Those who remain with their fathers risk being mistreated by their stepmothers, so they too seek refuge in towns or the city.

There has been a shift in marriage patterns. Many young couples are avoiding the formal and socially accepted type of marriage in favour of the "lesser" ones. Could the "lesser" form of marriage contribute to the increase in divorce as some interviewees claimed? Moreover, there is no room for admonition in the lesser forms of marriage, and neither the brides nor the grooms are admonished.

Divorce is not a problem among the Nyakusa only, for other societies in Tanzania face it too. Thus, there is a need for government, religious bodies, and civil society to educate people about the importance of tolerance in marriage.

Out-of-wedlock pregnancies are a new phenomenon to Nyakusa culture. Many people tend to blame them on education. What they fail to realize is that education raises the age of marriage, which is a positive development when we consider the health of girls and their newborns. It cannot, however, be disputed that because girls no longer marry before or at puberty, some of them are bound to misbehave and to fall pregnant. Rich men have a share of the blame for this issue. Some reasons advanced by respondents to out-of-wedlock pregnancies are, "girls' love of money" and "girls are cheated by men". There is a song about girls' love of money.

Song 4	*Njobela ea, aea he, hamba sosi* (twice)
	Imilumyana he, imilumyana gilekile ukuhaha sikuhaha
	sindalama aea ha, hamba sosi (twice)
	Njobela ea, aea he, hamba sosi (twice)
	Imilindwana he, imilindwana kigupija ga magege ga figane
	aea he, hamba sosi (twice)
Translation	Talk for me, ea, aea he hamba sosi
	Boys, eh, boys have stopped wooing. It is money that
	woos, aea he, hamba sosi
	Talk for me ea, aea he, hamba sosi
	Girls, eh, girls cook fish for the lovers, aea he,
	hamba sosi

The song relates how boys are no longer proposing to girls. Rather it is their money that proposes on their behalf. In response, girls cook fish and give it to their lovers. This song was sung many years after Song 1 above. By the time of Song 4, it was claimed that girls only went to men with money: in other words, true love no longer exists.

However, if girls were after money and no men responded, there would obviously be a reduction in out-of-wedlock pregnancies. On the other hand, many men make false promises of marriage and give gifts to girls who are deserted once they fall pregnant. Out-of-wedlock pregnancies is another issue that cuts across Tanzanian society. There is a need to educate girls to say "NO" whenever they are approached by ruthless men.

Sexuality among the Nyakusa has changed over the years. The disappearance of husband inheritance is good because girls are no longer bound to marry their sisters' or aunts' husbands. The fact that wife inheritance is dying out is encouraging because widows should have rights to marry whoever they want or not to marry at all. As to examination for virginity, just imagine a group of old women surrounding a 15-year-old teenager and demanding to see her vagina! I believe no one is mourning the death of a Nyakusa custom that is hostile to women, not least because only brides were examined while nothing was done to confirm that the bridegrooms were also "pure" upon first entering marriage.

A 70-year-old woman in Mbeya told us that when she was growing up all the girls were gathered and admonished. In those days, it was taken for granted that elders in the community would ensure that their children were well behaved. Any elder could admonish any child found misbehaving. This habit has disappeared and is deeply mourned. The result is that women and men interviewees associated "poor upbringing of the girls" with many current bad habits, such as out-of-wedlock pregnancies, increase in divorce rates, and disregarding the formal procedures of marriage. It is important that the Nyakusa revive this custom of admonition. It will put children back on the proper track. Boys too should be admonished, for they need to know how to behave especially now that AIDS is with us.

Gender sensitization

Having explored the changes that have take place in teenage sexuality among the Nyakusa, I suggest that *gender sensitization* seminars and

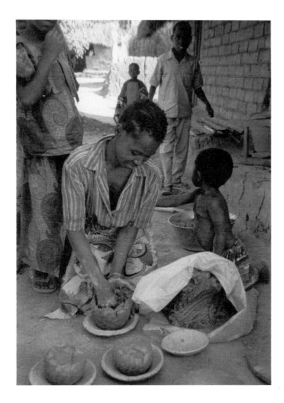

Income generation is undertaken by the wives for the
welfare of their families, husbands included.
(Photo Rita Liljeström)

courses should be conducted among Nyakusa men and women. In
this way, they will better understand their changing society and can
respond appropriately.

Gender sensitization of men

Men should be made aware that women are not undermining their
economic power. The need is there because, according to my findings,
women's participation in income generating activities, such as selling
secondhand clothes (*mitumba*) and bananas, worries husbands to the
extent that it can cause divorce. They should be made aware that income generation is undertaken by wives for the welfare of the families, husbands included. They should be informed that gender equality is a basic human right. They should not prevent women from
being educated out of subordination. Education has created
awareness among women of their fundamental rights. Men too have
to be educated so that the subordination of women dies out. Nyakusa

society should revise gender roles and readdress them so that gender equality can be attained. This recommendation arises from the fact that some respondents ascribed the increase in divorce and the persistence of wifely desertion to the education of women, who then rejected subordination.

Gender sensitization of women

Women should be sensitized to the fact that basic family needs are served when both women and men work. Thus, gaining access to money through income generation should not cause women to look down on their husbands. Income generating activities by women are analogous to farming by men, except that the money comes directly into the women's hands rather than their husbands'. They should also be sensitized into discussing their economic activities with their husbands. The need for sensitizing women exists because, according to the findings, it appears that women exult in their achievements to their husbands, or the husbands are jealous of their wives' achievements.

Gender sensitization of society

In the past, it was not possible for women to indulge in income generation because roads barely existed, and markets were beyond reach. On the other hand, men were in control of commercial crops such as coffee, hence their direct access to money. At present, both men and women have direct access to money because of economic development. This being the case, there is a need for men and women to treat each other with mutual respect so as to minimize divorce and desertion.

Society should realize that at present there are things which cannot be avoided. One of them is mixed marriages. These were nonexistent in the past because Bunyakusa was a closed society. Interaction among people from different tribes and nationalities has come with improvements in communication and transportation. Just as some Nyakusa marriages do not work out well so do some mixed marriages.

I am of the opinion that once the Banyakusa have been fully sensitized, families will be happier.

References

Bledsoe, C.H. and B. Cohen, 1993, *Social Dynamics of Adolescent Fertility in Sub-Saharan Africa*. Washington. DC: National Academy Press.

Charsley, S.R., 1969, *Princes of Nyakusa*. Nairobi: East African Publishing House.

Katapa, R.S., 1993, *Mother's Marital Status as a Correlate of Child Welfare in Tanzania*. Research report submitted to the Population Council, New York.

Wilson, G., 1936, "An introduction Nyakusa Society", *Bantu Studies X*.

1951, "The Nyakusa of South-Western Tanganyika", in E. Colson and M. Gluckman (eds.), *Seven Tribes of British Central Africa*. London: Oxford University Press.

—and M. Wilson, 1945, *The Analysis of Social Change: Based on Observations in Central Africa*. Cambridge: The University Press.

Wilson, M., 1950, "Nyakusa Kinship", in A.R. Radcliffe-Brown and Daryll Forde (eds.), *African Systems of Kinship and Marriage*. London: Oxford University Press for the International African Institute.

—1952, *Good Company*. London: Oxford University Press for the International African Institute.

—1957, *Rituals of Kinship among the Nyakusa*. London: Oxford University Press for the International African Institute.

—1959, *Communal Rituals of the Nyakusa*. London: Oxford University Press for the International African Institute.

—1970, *Rituals of Kinship among the Nyakusa*. Reprint. London: Oxford University Press for the International African Institute.

—1977, *For Men and Elders: Change in the Relations of Generations and of Men and Women amongst the Nyakusa-Ngonde People 1875–1975*. London: Oxford University Press for the International African Institute.

Chapter 3
The Erosion of the Matrilineal Order of the Wamwera

Mary Shuma and Rita Liljeström

In my previous study (Shuma, 1994), I focused on the problem of teenage pregnancies and early initiation. I was chiefly concerned with the conflicts between customary and modern education, arranged marriages, and the matrilineal system of the Wamwera.

The Wamwera are found in Lindi, one of the provinces of southern Tanzania. The region has a population of 646, 500, according to the 1988 census. The population is generally sparsely distributed, with a density of no more than 10 people per square kilometre. Soils are fairly poor and most people are subsistence farmers.

Ruangwa district was established in 1995. The district has about 150,000 in habitants. Ruangwa division contains thirty-one villages, and a population of 44,330 people. Ruangwa town consists of five squatter villages. Seventy-four to eighty per cent of the population is Muslim. The Muslim influence is very strong. The Wamwera combination of being Muslim and having a matrilineal background illustrates the marked ethnic diversity of the Tanzanian periphery.

This time, my aim is to tackle some of the questions that were not answered in my previous study. These include the erosion of matriliny and the destabilization of marriage as an institution. To gain insight into the current situation, one needs to understand how changes have developed over time. Therefore, I decided to interview elderly people in Lindi, people who grew up under the old order, but who have seen the matrilineal rules lose their validity.

I made two field trips to Lindi. On the second trip, Rita Liljeström joined me. We interviewed six elderly men (70 to 90 years), had a group discussion and some interviews with men between 40 and 68, and had interviews and talks with a handful of boys in their upper teens and early twenties. Why did we select men as our informants? The ambiguities in the obligations of a woman's maternal uncle and her husband seem to provoke and initiate change in the matrilineal system. We wanted to explore how these tensions are experienced by men. Secondly, after my earlier interviews with teenage girls, we now wanted to know more about the Wamwera men's point of view. However, I also add some evidence from women who are witnesses to or victims of the disintegration of old institutions.

About matriliny in Africa

The literature indicates that matrilineal societies are widespread in Africa. There is a matrilineal belt stretching all the way from Niger in North West Africa through Ghana, Nigeria, Benin, Zaire, Zambia, Malawi, Mozambique, and Tanzania.

Matrilineal ethnic groups had and still retain several features in common. They all trace their ancestry through common ancestries. They are matrilocal, which means that the groom resides with his wife and in-laws. Rites of passage are observed more strictly than in patrilineal societies and the woman and her kinsfolk have the right to inherit and bequeath property. Divorce rates also tend to be high and this is a longstanding characteristic rather than a recent development resulting from the introduction of cash economy.

In Tanzania, matrilineal groups that exist today are the Kaguru, Luguru, Zaramo, Makonde, Yao, Mwera, Makua, and Sagara. The Wamwera are discussed as part of a cluster of matrilineal societies examined by Hokororo (1961) in his work on the church at Lukuledi. According to him, the reason for examining the Wamwera in this context is that constant intermarriage and close social, political, and economic ties to other groups had resulted in the fusion of their particular customs, which no longer remained separate or distinct. They have similar beliefs and traditions and their reaction to Christian doctrine is similar to other tribes in the region.

According to Hokororo, marriage take places in the following four ways:

- arrangements are made by both sets of parents;
- by personal choice, but subject to the approval of parents and the maternal uncle;
- by cross-cousin marriages; and
- when a man inherits the widow of his brother.

Decisions are made in a context where the father is head of the domestic household and the maternal uncle is the overall head of the clan. He is referred to as the "keeper of the sisters" or the "owner of the sisters". Bridewealth is paid to the kin of the girl and the man goes through a period of testing to prove his loyalty and commitment to the family. If he meets the approval of the girl's maternal uncle and her kinfolk, then the marriage is legitimized by the giving of gifts and a final set of presents to the girl's kin.

Wamwera customs as related by elderly men

As informants we decided to use old men, who were initiated in 1920s and 1930s and who married shortly thereafter. Those men still remember their boyhood and initiation into manhood. They are all fathers and grandfathers, and some had numerous great-grand-children. Thus, they can testify about how Wamwera customs and conditions have been affected by the diverse forces and ideas of the twentieth century that were imposed on them.

Whereas it is Western custom to put emphasis on numbers, elderly Wamwera do not count or remember past events by years. Consequently, data on ages such as marital age, should not be taken literally. Ages are sometimes given simply to please foreign inter-viewers with their apparently superstitious interest in figures, as if they revealed secrets. Some obvious inconsistencies in ages may arise from a tendency to overstate or understate one's point in order to make it clear. When the interviewer is told that initiations today in-volve 4 to 5 year olds, this is a powerful way to illustrate the lowering of ages without necessarily being precise about age. By understanding the context, the interviewer is usually able to interpret the data as facts or trends.

The village elder

Mr. Chalira Mbene, 90 years, is the oldest man in Ruangwa. His hair is grey-white, as is his thin moustache. His face has several birthmarks. He is dressed in a white undershirt with long sleeves and sits on a wooden armchair stretching his legs forward. A long stick leans against the chair, ready to serve its master. His right leg is swollen and makes him less mobile. Mr. Mbene's eyes are keen and alive.

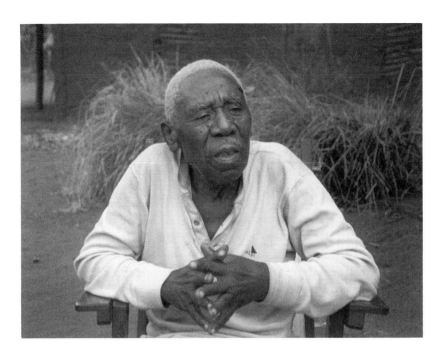

The village elder   (Photo Rita Liljeström)

Mr. Mbene is part of the living history of his country. As a boy, he lived under German rule, and later under the colonial rule of the British, and eventually in a country that achieved independence in 1961. Being of Wamwera origin, he has always lived in the same village, and although the village has moved, he has never been outside its social confines.

When he was young, the children in a family, boys and girls, worked together while their father or uncle instructed them about how to do the jobs around the homestead. They also taught them by saying: "Look around, we are here. This is our settlement. You should not go far away from us, and if you go, you have to tell us where you are going and why." And they reminded the children to "do the good, not the bad".

In examining the uncle and the father, who of them decides? Who has the last word? Mr. Mbene answers: "Father and mother are the starting point in life, the uncle and others just participate in discussion."

How was initiation in your boyhood?

Father and mother decide when the time is ripe for circumcision. They inform all the people, and the boys are told and invited. In the past, they were between 10 and 12 years of age. Old enough to understand what they were taught: how to do farming, as well as the moral values of Wamwera—to be polite, show hospitality, and be sincere. Teaching about marriage was at that time. However, they should not practise sexual intercourse before they were 20. One should not marry a person who was still a child. No marriage should take place soon after first menstruation.

Mr. Mbene himself married at 25 years of age. The marriage was first privately discussed between the uncle and the father. They chose the girl, who was 22 years, and he was offered to her. He paid ten shillings in bridewealth, according to the prevailing rate in the 1930s. This first wife bore him only two children before she died. In his second marriage all seven children died from different diseases. The surviving two from the first marriage, a daughter and a son, had eight children between them, and so far those eight have given him sixteen grandchildren. They in turn have lots of children of their own. They all live in Ruangwa, on the spot where we meet them. We are sitting inside a large homestead comprising several mudhuts with thatched roofs. Some houses are round, others square. There are papaya and mango trees. Around an outdoor kitchen several women and children are working or sitting and talking. These are grandchildren and daughters-in-law of his children. While we talk, an elderly woman sitting under a tree a few metres behind, listens. She is Mr. Mbene's second wife. I wonder what it is like to have lost seven children and to live in the midst of all those young mothers. I do not see her join the other women. She might be more interested in hearing what her husband tells a foreigner.

Considering the high marital age, were premarital relationships common in the past? "Yes, boys and girls had children before marriage, once they had reached adolescence." Did they marry then? "Few of them married. Others completely ignored the pregnancy. The parents of the girl took care of the child." Did premarital pregnancy have any impact on the future bridewealth of the girl? "It did not matter at all if you had a child or not, or if you had been married before." Why were the marriages so late? "There were fewer women than men. Furthermore, parents were very strict about the marital age, because only when young men's and women's brains have completed their growth, are they able to lead a better life. And it takes time before the brain is fully developed."

What was the role of the age-groups?

> Those of the same age were always gathered together. If the government raised any issue, they discussed it together. Wise men were selected to be their leaders. Everything concerning society must first be brought to the leader, and he brings it forth to the group. The same went for women. They took part in farming, initiation, celebration, and they prepared the local liquors.

How much bridewealth did you receive when you married your daughter off?

> I received fifty shillings for my daughter, and I paid sixty for my son's wife. The bridewealth for my granddaughter was 1,000 shillings, and 20,000 for my grandson's wife. All my granddaughters have a husband and nobody has divorced. However, five of my grandsons are not yet married although they have children. In fact, they are notorious for conceiving children out-of-wedlock. The money is not the problem. Nowadays, there is a surplus of women. It is not necessary to have a wife, there are women available everywhere.

> It should be the duty of the government to identify this issue and educate the society and undertake concrete measures. For the time being, since there are still old men alive, these men should meet the government and suggest various improvements to the government: primary schools, cinemas, and party celebrations should provide sex education. So far this is 100 per cent absent. There are no facilities to prevent early pregnancies. Sexual activity is there and can be suppressed no more, but there are no means for preventing pregnancies,

So says, Mr. Mbene, an old Muslim.

Did your son and daughter go through initiation. "Yes, the custom is still practised annually. I myself suggest the date."

Is the content of what is taught still the same?

> Although circumcision is undertaken, it happens in at an early age. Boys of four or five years know nothing. The boys have lost the idea of circumcision and its aims. They are not ready to marry. Nevertheless, they are sexually active and having children. The girls are not ready to get married. They receive the boys and conceive children with no assurance of support from the father. Boys and girls in these small towns are not prepared to do the farming. Old people cultivate the land although the young should take over. Economically this is destructive. The govern-

ment should be informed about how our customs have deteriorated and work towards a solution.

The sun has displaced the shadow. Mr. Mbene's answers are getting longer and more elaborate, whereas Mr. Sijale, the interpreter, is getting tired and his accounts are shorter and shorter.

The changes during your lifetime have been tremendous:

> In the past the German and British governments forced people to do jobs for the development of the colonial economy. If anyone had not paid his taxes he was in effect tortured by a system that did not care if there were droughts or floods. It was force without teaching about agricultural practices, cultivation without adequate technology. The death rates were high, people suffered from all kinds of diseases. The Germans were the worst.

> Still, we could overcome the Germans and British rule, but then came the *ujamaa* policies and their impact on the customs of Wamwera society. The establishment of the *ujamaa* villages meant that not only Wamwera customs but the clan itself dissolved. Before *ujamaa* we were living in groups with cashew-nut fields and enough fertile land around our homestead. Yet, we were moved far from our own place. We failed to maintain our fields and farms. Our unmanaged farms are three miles from here. On the other hand, the advantage of *ujamaa* was what we gained collectively: water, a hospital, schools, transport. And when a person died we could receive cash to bury the dead.

> At present, the advantages are the reverse of what was the case earlier. We know why we pay taxes. We know why we participate in self-help activities. Agricultural practices are taught, and we set our own priorities in farming.

We wanted to hear other opinions about the broad development topics that Mr. Mbene had touched on. A meeting with a local politician gave us an opportunity to do this. He is a retired teacher and a former CMM (*Chama cha Mapinduzi*, the ruling Revolutionary Party) party secretary and member of the district assembly. In fact, he joined CCM as party secretary in 1987. When we asked him to evaluate the changes that had taken place over the last ten years, he first mentioned the improvements in nutrition, housing, animal husbandry, and then moved on to what has gone wrong in social and cultural life:

> The material aspects of life have improved whereas some other aspects have worsened. The deterioration of Wamwera tribal custom has meant a great loss concerning children. The Wamwera were living in groups with a common homestead. There the children were taught Wamwera cul-

ture—how to help each other and their parents. They became familiar with Wamwera values about hospitality and the danger of using bad language. All these things were simple. Twenty years back the maternal uncle was obliged to help his nephews. But no longer. The establishment of *ujamaa* villages led to detrimental changes. People with bad manners and different beliefs were mixed with people who followed their customs. As a result, the moral order of the Wamwera eroded, and the bonds between generations have weakened.

There are better roads and new people move in and out. Young boys and girls are not afraid of moving to Dar es Salaam, Nairobi, and other distant places. They even go without asking permission. Cinemas, the good ones and the ugly ones, radiocasettes and music, have swept away the world view of the Wamwera.

The children are split into two groups, those who are anxious about getting an education, and those who do not care about education. No wonder; those teacher who now retire were committed, the new groups of teachers are not. This bad situation has existed for the past few years. Some teachers are not qualified and not committed. In such conditions, school just means wasting time. The youth choose to join self-reliance projects instead.

Mzee Chani

Mzee Chani is seated on a locally made wooden chair. Together with him, seated on a mat, are his wife and several relatives. He is chewing green boiled pigeon peas, locally known as *mikumbu*, while his relatives prepare green pigeon peas for cooking. Although Mzee Chani cannot tell his age, he remembers to having been born in 1916, which meant he is about 78 years old. Unfortunately, Mzee Chani cannot see anymore. He lost his eyesight five years back, and confesses he has been able to survive only thanks to the care of his wife, who appears much younger than him. Mzee Chani is a man of wisdom and he narrates his experience as a Mwera as follows:

> I was born at Mtenga and was first washed by waters from Mtenga. My father got engaged *(kulomba)* to my mother, when she was still very young. She was not mature yet; neither had she been initiated. Since traditional marriage was conducted at the bride's place, the couple automatically went to live there. This is what happened to my father—he had to move to my mother's homestead after engagement. Since his wife, my mother, was too young, my father was required to move to Mnancho until the bride got older. When the bride was old enough and had gone through initiation rites (locally known as *kuaruka unyago*) her parents accepted the bridewealth, which was in the form of cloth remnants and a

locally made gun (*gobole*). The customary marriage was conducted at the bride's place and the couple lived with the bride's parents. All the children born to my father and mother were born at her parents' place. We are eight in total. I come seventh. My parents remained married into old age. Only a few years ago they died. Before they died, I arranged for a Christian marriage in order to get them blessed by the priest.

As a Roman Catholic I studied and taught in a church. I got married in 1938 aged 22. I do not remember the age of my first wife, but she had already gone through initiation ceremonies. *Kuaruka* is one of the requirements for one to get married. It applies to both boys and girls. I married and lived with my in-laws. After some time, my parents arranged for me to go and live with them. My first wife gave me four children, but now only a daughter remains. The other three died. My only daughter was born 1938, the same year that I married her mother.

Another point Mzee Chani stressed was the role of parents and maternal uncles in the marriages of children. He mentioned that both the parents and maternal uncles chose the spouses of both boys and girls. The implication is that they well knew the tastes of their children and the kind of spouses from the community who would make for happy marriages. Thus, the chances that the children would object to the choice of spouse was minimized and rarely occurred. For a girl or a boy to object to the spouse chosen by parents and maternal uncles was seen as a bad omen for the young person. Such arranged marriages lasted longer than modern marriages.

Had my former wife agreed to move with me to the new business area, Lukwika, I would not have married another wife. But since she refused to move from her parents' premises, I had no alternative but to marry another wife. Yet that did not mean divorce. We still remain husband and wife even in separation.

I married this one (pointing to his wife seated next to him) to take care of me. I have no children by her. Neither sets of parent's elders would wish to see one marry outside the community. They prefer marriage between families sharing the same matrilineal values and having a good relationship. The girl to be married was expected to be decent, and not have associated with men.

Earlier marriages involved faithfulness between the bride and groom and bridewealth entailed a token amount of cash, if any. Faith and trust between married couples is what kept marriages going. These days there is neither faith nor trust between married couples. Some marriages are arranged by the parents for monetary reasons. They do not care about marriage permanency. Children no longer belong to the maternal uncle's lineage. In our days, the maternal lineage played a big role in children's upbringing. Children inherited from their uncles. Things have changed.

My only daughter went to boarding school at a mission centre to study domestic science. The church elders wanted her to be a Catholic nun but I protested because I wanted her to marry and have children to expand our family. This was important as I had no children by my second marriage. I preferred a farmer to marry my daughter because a farmer settles on land and my grandchildren will be assured of land to farm and inherit.

My son-in-law-to-be, himself a farmers, came and lived with me in hope of marrying my daughter while she was still at boarding school. The son-in-law-to-be engaged in various family activities, and lived in my house. Arrangements for marriage were made by his parents. Food and local brew was prepared in my house. The marriage took place in a church but the celebrations took place in my house.

The newly married couple lived with me for quite awhile, until the groom's parents came to negotiate to take them to their house. I had no objection. They left, but later the man took paid employment as a police officer. He is currently retired and lives in another village. They have a total of ten children by their marriage. One died while still young and my daughter has stopped having more children on health grounds.

Asked whether he was happy that his daughter bore so many children, and whether his clan has been expanded, he said:

> Well I am happy, although things have changed. Children in this society are no longer named after the maternal clan. Therefore, some of her children have been given my name but not named after our clan. However, I am happy my daughter bore so many children. I am sure she is also happy.

While Mzee Chani spoke of the importance of decency among girls before marriage, it was strange to me that he made no reference to virginity as a precondition of marriage. Nevertheless, he stressed that a girl was expected to behave well and not to associate with men. This is as close that he came to mentioning virginity.

> However, in time fathers wanted to support their own children, who would receive little or no assistance from their maternal uncles. Paternal relatives have taken over. Children belong more and more to their biological fathers who play a parental role in their upbringing and in their marriages. There are no marriage consultations concerning our children anymore. They meet, love each other, and marry without the consent of their parents. They just inform the parents of their wish to get married or they just marry. They marry outside our locality, resulting in a mixture of cultures. Sometimes they marry within their own clan *(chipinga)*. Some par-

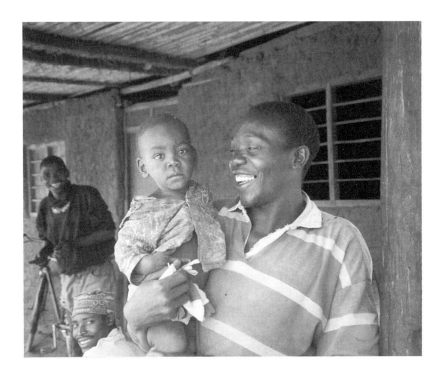

By time fathers equally wanted to support   (Photo Rita Liljeström)
their own children, who would receive little
or no assistance from their maternal uncles.

ents, on the other hand, push their daughters into marriage for what they
can get as bridewealth. Marriages no longer take our traditions, customs,
and values into consideration. Divorce rates are high. Some marry today
and after a month they divorce.

Mrs Chani. obviously shared her husband's opinions. She remained
seated beside her husband while he narrated his experience. Given the
opportunity to express her views, she said:

> Formerly marriages were more meaningful and more respected than
> these days. A girl would be identified and engaged by a man, but would
> never have sexual intercourse with him until they got married. Mzee, my
> husband, wants to report the initiates, who recently made a lot of noise
> and used obscene language, to the village council. I would suggest, if it
> was possible that these rites entail respect for religion. The young
> initiates should, among other things, be taught how to pray, and lead a
> Christian or Islamic life. It would be better than the obscene words they
> use throughout the night.

Both Mzee Chani and his wife illustrate in their views the significant impact that religion has had on traditional values among Wamwera. The fact that Mzee Chani was not content with his parents' customary marriage and arranged a Christian marriage for them says something about the role of the church in either damaging or improving people's attitudes. His action called customary marriage into question despite the government's recognition of the same. Yet he appears to be caught up in a social dilemma. He sees old Wamwera marriages as lasting longer than modern marriages, which, according to him, are often short-lived. It is not clear how he resolves this contradiction?

Another aspect which emerges from the Chani's views is the economic one. The traditional role of parents vis-à-vis the maternal uncle's involvement in the upbringing of children is changing. Maternal uncles are more conscious now of the economic burden that accompanies traditional responsibilities. They would rather spend more on their own children than on their sisters' children. Similarly, parents are unwilling to part with some of the bridewealth from their daughters for the sake of maternal uncles, especially if the uncles have not contributed to the upbringing of their nieces. Underlying all this is the tendency of parents to commercialize marriage. Bridewealth is no longer a token to publicly signify that the couples are now wife and husband. In the same way, the commercialization of land and economic activities has weakened the ties of community or family to land and has led to a redefinition and reconceptualization of the traditional economy.

Samuel Chimolo

Samuel Chimolo was born in 1905 and is now an old man under the care of his son, Munyuku. He is a short but energetic man seated in a wooden chair. He appears excited to be told that he was one of those chosen for an interview and he expresses his excitement thus: "This makes me an important man not only in my community but in Tanzania. Look at the lady; she has come all the way from Dar es Salaam looking for me."

During the interview, Chimolo had the following to tell:

> I spent three years in a mission school. I married a girl by the name of Ulusula. She is now deceased. It was my eldest sister who arranged for my marriage because my mother died while we were young. Ulusula was 18 years when I married her; while I was 23. There was no bride-

wealth. In my time, if one was working, could till the land well, and displayed an ability to work or produce independently, it was easy to get a woman in marriage. I had all the qualities mentioned, so it did not take long before my in-laws confirmed my marriage to Ulusula. The marriage entailed my moving to live with the in-laws. I lived with my in-laws for a short while and later built myself this small hut where I moved to live with my wife. My wife died in 1975. I decided not to marry another.

During her first pregnancy, Ulusula went through another initiation rite called *litiwa*. She gave me two children, both boys. The boys are now married. The first boy married at 18 and his bride was 16 years old, but the bride could not conceive until the age of 19. They had a total of nine children—two died at a tender age. The second boy married about the same age as his elder brother and has a total of seven children. Both my sons are now grandfathers. In the course of their marriage, bridewealth was paid. It was a small, token amount of cash, equivalent probably to the present (1996) value of 300 to 400 shillings. They consulted me or my brother before they got married. Their maternal uncle was not involved because he did not take part in their upbringing.

Both my children are married and live with their wives in the houses they constructed. The idea of moving to live with the in-laws did not apply to them as things had changed by the time they got married. Naming children after maternal uncles is no longer practised. Children belong to the mother and biological father. Everybody has responsibility for his or her children's upbringing. It is only when the maternal uncle has played a part in the upbringing of his sisters' children that those children are named after him. Even my own sister's children are currently named after their father.

Of his own experience with regard to Wamwera marriage, Chimolo observed:

> Maternal relatives are responsible for marriage affairs among the Wamwera. Parents of both parties meet to discuss and decide on bridewealth which could be in the form of cash, a token, or in kind (a hen, handhoe, axe, etc.). The bridewealth to be given would be agreed upon to satisfy the bride's family. They would share the bridewealth among parents and uncles, so that it could be repaid in case of divorce. Earlier marriages involved movement of the groom to live with the bride at his in-law's. Children born to such marriages were named after maternal uncles. There are very few people currently doing this: a majority of us have dropped this tradition. As long as a person showed an ability to work and produce independently, marriage would not be denied.

On the question of who brought him up, he replied: "I am called Chimolo, after my mother's clan. In fact, my father's name, Nnunduma, comes from his mother's clan. However, my sister's children are currently named after their fathers. Names go with the one who takes care of the children.

Three issues emerge from Chimolo's views. One is the significance of being self-reliant. A boy was able to marry if he proved self-reliant. The girl's maternal uncles, together with her brothers, were certifiers of this characteristic, for the groom lived and worked for and with them. A dependent boy was not ready to support his wife and children and could not, therefore, marry.

The second is the collective responsibility inherent in the matter of naming children among the Wamwera. The sharing of bridewealth among maternal uncles and the bride's actual parents spread the risk and ensured that many relatives assumed responsibility for whatever mishaps that might befall the bride in future. This was collective responsibility which none could escape.

The third issue concerns the way in which children carried names from their mother's clan to ensure the continuity of the matriliny and downplay patriliny. This is seemingly empowerment of women. However, all decision-making powers remained the exclusive domain of a girl's or woman's brothers and maternal uncles. In the presence of brothers, sisters had no more say in matters that affected them than a wife did in the presence of her husband or her father.

However, there is an tendency to abandon the custom of naming children after the mother's clan. For example, Mr. Atonda, an elderly farmer, stated that he had changed from the maternal to the paternal line in naming his children:

> I do not regard it important to keep the mother's line. In my opinion, the power should go to the male side. When I was a boy, the maternal uncle still had power, whereas after I grew up and considered the issue, I told my wife that our children would take the name from my side, my maternal name. She agreed. Her maternal uncles did not take any action. I was independent in my own house.

> Such changes have become more common around here. I know about five families who have decided to follow the paternal line, although most families stick to the uncle's name.

The three principal male informants all commented on signs of erosion of Wamwera customs, especially that the maternal uncle no longer has the obligations which he used to discharge in the past, like bringing up his sister's children and taking part in arranging their marriages. Fathers and parental relatives have taken over. They, like the maternal uncles, prefer to spend more on their own children than on their sisters children. Consequently, the children are no longer named after their maternal clan. Neither did the practice of moving to live with the in-laws apply to the old men's children.

Even institutions like initiation and marriage have lost their former meaning. The initiation age has been lowered and the young boys are not ready to shoulder the duties of manhood. Mr. Mbene's grandsons are not married, although they have children. According to their grandfather, they are notorious for conceiving children out-of-wedlock. Similar opinions and experiences were expressed by most of our informants over 50. Consequently, we looked closer at current initiation and marriage practices.

Initiation into manhood

About 75 years ago, when Mr. Mbene was a young boy, the peer-group of initiates was instructed about farming, Wamwera moral values, and the obligations that followed from marriage. Contrariwise, today young boys have lost the real meaning of circumcision and its aims. They are not ready to marry. Nevertheless, they are sexually active and conceive children. Such comparisons between the past and present were common in our interviews, the message being that things were better in the past.

> In our day initiation was delayed until one became engaged, when the girl was initiated for marriage. Today that is no longer the case. These days, immediately a child is initiated she or he starts playing at sex, a result of which is early pregnancy and sometimes maternal deaths.

Now and then people refer to the commercialization of social life. Mr. Natondo observes:

> Initiation cannot be practised before the boys are 15 years. When younger boys and girls are brought along they do not understand anything. Today the boys and girls do not intend to live together in marriage. They look for relationships without permanence. They destroy their lives and catch various diseases. They need to be educated. Long ago, they were better prepared for life than they are at present. However, if today's parents tell them about the past, their children say that all that has passed and that they live according to the current conditions in the world. "You did as you did because you were not civilized."

> Changes in circumcision came about when mothers and fathers began to invite lots of people and serve local beer. Initiation became a business, a part of the economy. The guests contributed money. It was no longer taken seriously, and people no longer bothered about the age of the boys.

A retired civil servant, Mr. Martin Kabona, named Kabona from his maternal side, went through initiation at the age of 9 years. The circumcision was conducted by traditional medicine men. He stayed in the forest for three months. During that time, his group was oriented into adulthood, by a man chosen by their families The man was to look after the boys' health, to cook for them, train them for good conduct, and give them instruction about marriage. After three months, the boys would graduate as adults and marriage would be allowed so that they could start a family, as well as get help for farming. The boys were also expected to follow clan traditions and restrictions. For example, if a man had an expectant wife, he would not put on a shirt. By following the rules, one could safeguard the pregnancy.

Kabona sees initiation of both boys and girls as having lost its principal meaning. These days, initiation stresses that one has become an adult, even at such a tender initiation age of 7 or 8 years, and is ready for marriage. Initiation is, therefore, encouraging early free sex among youngsters. It is also contributing to the youngsters' lack of interest in continuing with school, especially among girls. It is expected that a girl who passed through initiation is not a virgin, because initiation encourages sex.

Kabona sees a radical change in the meaning that initiation has for boys. Initiation was meant to make a boy self-reliant. Almost 85 per cent of the worthwhile purpose of initiation has gone. He explains:

> The costs of sending young boys for initiation have escalated, while schooling has contributed to changes in the age of initiation. Parents have consequently lowered the initiation age to 7 or 8 to reduce the cost of caring for the initiates, including buying new clothes for graduation. I am sure that what the boys are taught during initiation does not make much sense for them because of their tender age. People are conducting initiation just for the sake of it. Some things are postponed, but then never communicated at all since there is no further initiation. With all the visitors to Ruangwa and a lot of intermarriage, I suspect that initiation will continue to lose its real meaning.

We were aware that children were initiated before they started school because the school did not permit the children to stay away while participating in initiation rites. The authorities have even imprisoned a Mwera father who allowed his daughter to be away from school during the months of initiation and seclusion. This conflict between traditional and modern preparation for life ended in victory for the

modern. Initiation has to take place at a pre-school age to avoid inter-
ference with school.

This approach has also entailed some benefits:

> The initiation ceremony for a young child is cheaper than for an older
> one—especially as far as his clothing requirements are concerned. Parents
> are, therefore, rushing their children to initiation because of the lower
> costs of their ceremonies as well as because of the school requirements.

I remember that, while talking to Mrs. Chani I had heard boys singing
in the distance. She commented:

> You hear those boys sing? They are on the initiation course. These days
> initiation centres are located at places where the people live. In the past,
> they used to take boys to a forest far from the settlements. They could,
> therefore, not be heard or seen until they came out of the forest. These
> ones make a noise throughout the night. Last night we could not sleep
> because of their obscene (*matusi*) language. The kind of words these very
> young boys use, is unbearably pathetic. I dare not repeat them to you.
> They are purely obscene. What kind of adults will such initiates become?
> The essential meaning of initiation is dying out.

Mrs. Chani brought up another aspect of change arising from environmental threats to traditional practices. The large forests which
suited customary initiation have been cleared for crop cultivation and
can no longer seclude the initiates. What used to be strict secrets are
now revealed in the open and the inherent myths and symbols that
went with those secrets are laid bare. No wonder there are questions
about and deviance from symbols whose origin and meaning are not
understood.

Can formal schooling absorb some of the ideals behind the practices and discard the unnecessary ones? There seems to be no about-
turn. When do *matusi* (obscene words) become *matusi*? Is it when they
are heard by people who are not, because of their age, supposed to
hear them? Why should words, which are freely uttered by everyone
who goes (or went) through initiation rites, later turn into *matusi*?

The young boys' experiences

After listening to the alarmed views of elderly people, I wanted to talk
to some young boys about initiation and their sexual relationships.
Mr. Kabona volunteered to escort me to interview some of the boys.
We first went to Likangare Primary School where I met 17-year-old

Juma Maulo. He was initiated at the age of 7. However, he recently began to take a girl to bed. She is his age mate and they went through initiation at the same time. So far they have not considered any measures to prevent pregnancy. Juma is thinking about it. He was 7 years old at initiation, the lowest age among the boys I interviewed.

In what follows, three boys share their experiences about initiation. The first one is 16-year-old Vituku Salomo. He is still in school, currently in Standard 6:

> I went for circumcision at the age of 9. I went through various stages: All the hair on my head was removed a day before and at night I was taken to *viwanjani*, a place where circumcision is to be performed. At the *viwanjani*, old men came to invoke the ancestors, praying for safe circumcision for all of us. Traditional dancing goes on the whole night. It is performed by the owner of the *viwanjani* and his group. The dance before circumcision is called *mkomanga*. Next day, in the afternoon the *ngariba* executes the circumcision. It is called *kuaruka*. The *ngariba* cuts a piece of skin from our male organ. Then he applies traditional medicine and ties it with a bandage. We are then left in the forest for one-and-a-half months until each of us has healed completely.
>
> While in the forest, we listened to a lot of teachings by *walombo*. They are guardians chosen by our parents to care for us in the forest. They taught us good behaviour, how to behave as adults, clan proscriptions, including "not to open the mother's pot; not to go into the mother's sleeping room without permission, etc.". Each *mlombo* would care for an average of two boys. The *walombo* are chosen for their good behaviour and they are supposed to be forceful young men. Sometimes they are paid a token amount.
>
> Our return from the forest is marked by a big ceremony and dance called *kiangubo*. Upon our return, we put tree bark around our waists. This is called *manguanga*. We join the dance while wearing *manguanga*, and in the afternoon our bodies are washed. The washing involves an aunt lying on the ground while one steps on her back and is washed while standing on her. Normally it is another aunt or sister who is supposed to wash us. After the washing, new clothes are brought, put on you and you are carried around the dancing ground either by the *mlombo* or your mother. While the ceremony continues, a group of women bring traditional medicine, *dawa ya unyago*, and apply that to one and the other boys for protection. Gifts are given, including token gifts. The first night is spent out with the *walombo*, but later we move to the house to sleep.

So far Vituku has not had any relationship with a girl.

Pambo Kambona is a Primary 7 pupil, aged 18. He went for initiation at the age of 8.

Initiation is the tradition observed by our ancestors, hence I regard it as a necessity of life. Early preparations are done, and the *ngariba* is chosen by parents according to his experience in performing circumcision. The *ngaribas* are paid by parents. I was laid down on my back; one strong man held my legs, another my arms. *Ngariba* takes a sharp knife and cuts the protruding skin on my organ, while he later uses his special long finger nail to peel off the rest of the skin. The peeling is done twice before the skin is finally cut. It is extremely painful, but one is expected not to scream. A traditional healer brings some medication, applies it to the bleeding wound, and a cloth rag is used as a bandage for the wound. The cutting knife is not washed but later the traditional healer sprays some medicine, similar to maize flour, on it. Later he wipes the knife and keeps it. This is the way it is done. After cutting everybody, the *ngariba* runs to the waiting parents to break the news that each boy has been circumcised.

We are kept in the forest for a period of no less than a month, until everyone has healed. *Walombo* take care of us, washing us, cooking and feeding us, etc. Among the things our *mlombo* told us was that we should "not to go to bed with a girl who has not been initiated". This is forbidden in our tradition, and if one does it, one is ostracized, and if a girl who has not been initiated falls pregnant, the offspring is killed. Again, we were forbidden to talk about initiation to those who have not gone through it yet. Each *mlombo* is free to communicate as much information as he wishes. My *mlombo* went on to forbid me from disturbing my parents when they are in their bedroom. He told me how to care for a pregnant woman and a baby.

I had my first sexual encounter after initiation, but I had not yet become a man (had not released semen). I had the encounter in the wilderness with a girl of my age. I am no longer in touch with her. I do not remember enjoying it. I released semen in 1995 and ever since I have gone to bed with various girls. I would say that I have enjoyed sex and it feels great. I have sex with girls in our house. I meet my current girl two or three times a week.

James is 21 years. He could not finish Class 7 because he had made a schoolgirl pregnant, and hence was thrown out of school. Currently a farmer, he grows maize and cassava. He is temporarily living with the girl he made pregnant. They have a 2-year-old girl.

James was initiated at the age of 10 years, but in the mission:

It was, therefore, a medical person who circumcised me and not a traditional *ngariba*. After circumcision, we were put up into a hut next to the church, where a Catholic priest used to come and teach us how to respect our elders, especially our parents. Some traditional restrictions were explained to us by the priest, including, not going into the parents' bedroom, not to uncover your mother's pot, etc. Only medicine from the hospital was applied to my wound, including antibiotics. I was not treated with any traditional medicine since I did not go to the forest.

I never went to bed with a girl before initiation. In 1993, I had nocturnal dreams. In July the same year, I had my first intercourse. It was with a peer-group girl. I felt so good that I wanted to repeat it again and again. The girl had already been initiated and had experienced monthly periods. We continued the relationship for six months an had occasional sexual intercourse, but she did not fall pregnant. We used to meet anywhere in the bush.

Thereafter, I had sexual encounters with several others, until I met the mother of my kid. She was then 13 years old and I was 19. It was not long before she broke the news that she was pregnant. I am keeping her and the kid, but have not decided to marry her. I have another girlfriend away from here. We meet often. My child's mother has been enrolled in the family planning programme. Thus she is on contraceptives, but my girlfriend is not. I have used condoms. However, they are not readily available. I do not use condoms with my current girlfriend.

The initiation rites described by Vituku and Pambo appear serious and customary. Obviously, they made an impact on the boys. Vituku is the only one who had not yet had sexual relationship. It seems that once the boys become sexually active, they involve themselves in multiple relationships. Although all the boys had heard about HIV/AIDS on radio and had been taught about it in school, they do not take any precautions. The have the same dismissive attitudes towards contraception. James, the oldest of the boys, was circumcised at the mission hospital. Nonetheless, this modern method was combined with some customary teachings. However, the boy did not learn how to prevent pregnancies. He still takes risks with his girlfriend that he keeps in addition to the young mother of his daughter.

How do the interviews conducted with a handful of boys correspond with the descriptions given by the elderly men? The initiation, although at lower age and of shorter duration than in the past, seemed more intact and dignified than we expected. Yet it was not followed by marriages, although it prepared the boys for sexual manhood. What the boys relate confirms to a certain extent the concerns of the elderly that grandsons conceive children without any intention of marrying. Even if it is not true for all of them, some boys do lack trustworthiness and judgment in the way they act in manhood.

Our curiosity about changes in the institution of marriage had been whetted. We try to explore the topic further in the next two sections.

Weakening of Wamwera marriage

We arrived in Ruangwa in the late afternoon. The public offices were closed and all rooms at the government guesthouse were occupied. We spent the night at a local hotel near the market place. Inside the hotel there was an open space surrounded by several small sleeping stalls. The shower and the toilets were on the opposite side. After occupying a stall each, we were left to the voices and noises of the night. We found ourselves in the middle of a lively and loud sex trade. Lorries and traders stopped outside and young women from the village gathered around the hotel. We lay and listened to the negotiations which set the terms of trade between the women and their customers. Women giggled and men argued in hoarse and pressing voices. Occasionally, a fierce quarrel broke out. Now and then, wild laughter rent the night. Sometimes, the voices seemed so close as to be inside the room, sometimes they faded away into the distance.

Next day, while visiting the local restaurant and the market place, we observed how newcomers to the village, truck drivers and traders, were the object of assiduous attention by local women, who wanted to make assignations for the next night. Sexual services seemed to be one of the few avenues available to many women for generating cash, and demand is high. Next night, when we boarded at another guesthouse where government officials boarded, we slept deeply. Here the traffic was more discreet and longstanding guests had their semi-permanent and silent girlfriends. There were always people who liked to gossip and share their observations about their customers sleeping partners.

Roadside talk with a group of men

Mr. Sijale, an agricultural officer from the district office, acted as guide and interpreter. We went to a subdivision of the town and to a place where many people were assembled. There were some market stalls on an open space. Young mothers sat with their infants on long wooden benches. Young men were lounging around. Mr. Sijale introduced us to them all and explained why we were there. The young men became excited and started to make jokes about "changes in sexuality and marriage among the Wamwera" by using body language. One of them ate a banana in an obscene way, sucking on it and moving it in and out of his mouth, to the laughter of the others.

Mr. Sijale introduced me to Hamisi Mahoya, Mzee Mhulima, and Saidi Posho. They are Wamwera elders, about a generation younger than the old men we had interviewed previously, the youngest being 57 and the oldest 68 years. They all refused to be interviewed alone, but participated willingly when allowed to stay together.

I inquired for awhile about Wamwera customs and their changes, including maternal uncles and fathers. While Mr. Posho's father still moved to his mother's and his in-laws' place, married women nowadays move to the husband's homestead. We talked about initiation and manhood. Two men joined in explaining *unyago:* "After having been circumcized, the boys are called men. They are now expected to be sexually active, or at least this was the meaning of the ritual in the past."

Did you receive any instruction about how to act when approaching a woman? "It is not necessary to give practical instruction about intercourse—it will happen by itself. It comes automatically when the boy meets a girl. This happens regularly."

The group of elderly men now totals five. New men have joined our group and they all want to testify about their experiences. They discourage all curious listeners by shouting at them. People immediately obey them. Nobody disturbed us though we sat on common ground near the roadside.

> During the month of seclusion, the boys and the girls slept together, and they talked as if they were pairs. However, the sexual act was never completed.

Were you taught how to satisfy a woman?

A long discussion went on, and when it ended one of the men explained: "It should be an agreement. The woman should not be forced to have sex. A boy should not be that afraid of a woman that he cannot reach an agreement with her." One of the men thought that women learned more about how to satisfy a man, than vice versa. The other men agreed.

In the past, when they were young, sexual activity began before 18, while at present boys start sex at 15. The men had all married for the first time between the ages of 20 to 23, and their wives had been between 20 and 25. Two of the men had paid 15 shillings in bridewealth, while two men had paid 120 and 200 shillings respectively.

Two of the men have been married four times and had experienced three divorces. One of the two has ten children, seven living and three dead. The other one had lost only one of his eight children. Two men have married three times and divorced twice. One of them has two children, the other has had seven, but four of them have died. I do not know how many times the fifth man had divorced, but even he had a history of divorce.

The men had paid bridewealth even for their later marriages. One of them explained the custom by saying that "When you marry into another place, you start afresh and must pay the same."

Who receives the bridewealth?

> The bridewealth is collected by the woman of the bride's father. The relatives of the wife and bride's father will come together. The bride's mother—the mother-in-law, tells how much she has received and divides it equally among both sides—her own side and her husband's side. It has always been like that and it is still so today.

Where do the children stay after divorce? "Usually the children remain with the woman. In rare cases they stay with the father."

In the case of the men present, their children stayed with their mothers. However, one of the men adds: "The new wife of the father does not look after his earlier children. When the children are cared for by their mother, she will talk to the father if there is any problem."

Have all of you married mothers in your subsequent marriages? "Yes, it is true. When we married another wife, she usually had two or three children. We had to provide for her children. We cannot escape that by any means at all."

Why did you divorce? What reasons did you have for breaking up your marriages?

> The practice of polygamy or infidelity comes about because the first wife uses rude language, she is not willing to do the farming and cooking, and not ready to respond to her husband's needs. Since income depends on farming, the husband does not increase his wealth ranking enough, so he looks for other women.

One man says that he divorced his wife as her character was not good enough for him. The next man had troubles with his wife's relatives as he was not able to pay the remaining 20 shillings of bridewealth immediately. Two of the men had lived outside the region for years. When one eventually returned to Ruangwa, he and his wife decided to part. When the other husband came back home, he found that his wife was impressed by another man: "When I discovered that I had to let her marry him." All of you have married and remarried. Some people cohabit without marrying. What difference does it make? Mzee Muhlima explains:

> There are two main reason for cohabitation. One is that the partners have different religions. Secondly, even if they are of the same religion, they may reach a compromise over marriage. One comes to live with the other. They can stay for long and even have children. There are lots of such cases.

Did it ever happen that you abused your wife? One of the five says:

> If she is lazy and does not show respect, in such a situation she is first of all told and taught about her mistakes. If she does not correct herself, I will move out without telling her. I move out to marry another wife.

This answer is regarded as exhausting the topic.

People say that young men do not want to marry today? "One has to consider two issues. There are more girls than boys here. Furthermore, the boys do not feel ready to marry even if they have money. There are girls available anyhow."

If you were young today, would you prefer to marry or do like the young men do today?

> Big changes have taken place since we were young. In my opinion it is a must for a man to have a wife. If you are single, life is not complete. We all say that there are many things only a woman can do. A complete man ought to have a wife. Besides it is dangerous to jump from one woman to another (because of AIDS).

Here are the ages of each of the five men and the age of each of their latest wives: 65/39, 63/35, 57/29, 64/36, and 68/34. The age difference between the spouses spans over 26 to 34 years. The men have married women of their daughter's generation. In fact, their wives are almost age-mates of their granddaughters.

The pattern that emerges from our talk is this: young men make their girlfriends pregnant and then leave them, thus creating a pool of single mothers who look for male support. The old men's need for "completeness" and the single mother's need for support fit together.

How does the insecurity of marriage affect women?

The impact of socioeconomic change among the Wamwera and the contradictions it has created are highlighted in the narration of Sabina Chalamanda, a middle-aged Mwera woman. She is married and has been blessed with two children, a girl and a boy in their early teens. In many ways, she would be regarded a lucky woman to have managed to produce two replacements for herself and her husband. Yet Sabina does not consider herself lucky. Two children are perceived to be too few to raise her status among the Wamwera. Sabina's basic question is, to whom do Wamwera children belong? Who is actually responsible for them?

Let us have first-hand information from Sabina herself:

> I was brought up by a maternal uncle who played a big role in my marriage. In the course of my marriage, a hen or a token worth about 200 shillings was given to my uncle but that was just enough to call the relatives together to inform them of my marriage. The wedding was half-traditional and half-modern, in the sense that the ceremony was in a church but the all other activities were conducted according to Wamwera tradition. I am married to a Mwera man and have had only two children by him. I feel bad that I have been unable to bear more children. I had four miscarriages, and I lost my first three children at an early age before having these two, a son and a daughter. Since traditionally children belonged to the mother and the maternal side, I am responsible for my children's upbringing. I have constructed myself a simple mudhouse to which I will retire. That is my own house, and my husband does not care about it because I am obliged to take care of the children. Things have changed and maternal uncles are no longer there for their sisters' children. My husband still takes advantage of the society's attitude that children belong to mothers and maternal uncles, so he has not assisted me in the children's upbringing. I suspect he has children somewhere else because I have been unable to bear him more children.
>
> I would wish that my daughter get married at a later age, when she is working and independent so that she is capable of looking after her children in case of divorce. Divorce in this community is inevitable nowadays. Sometimes I ask myself whether marriages are at all important anymore. Yet, I would wish her to be married to a man from our tribe so

that we could conduct the traditional ceremonies together. If she married an outsider, she would find it difficult to cope with the traditions and I would see her infrequently.

It is no wonder that Sabina feels ambivalent about marriage. She is probably correct to point to the advantage her husband takes of the uncle's customary obligations towards his sisters' children. During the transitional phase in the transfer of obligations from the maternal uncle to the husband, the father of the child, it seems that both the men shirk their part by claiming that it is the other's responsibility. It appears to be a paradox that women are expected to give their husbands many children, while some husbands do not hesitate to abandon their wives and children.

Wamwera marriage in the past

In the early days, all Wamwera marriages followed custom. There were no Christian or Islamic marriages. Customary marriages involved arrangements by the parents. When the bride-to-be was identified by the groom, his maternal uncle and his parents would team up with the bride's family for marriage negotiations. After they reached the necessary agreements, marriage would take place. Girls used to be married even before menarche. The husband would move to his bride's homestead, although there would be no sexual relations until the onset of his wife's menarche. Instead, he would be given a separate hut to live in. The bride was expected to announce the onset of menarche so that she and her husband could start having sexual intercourse. From the day they were allowed to sleep together, three big logs (*magogo*) of *mninga*, firewood, would be used to prepare food—both stew and stiff porridge (*mchuzi na ugali*). *Mninga* was used because it is a hard-wood that burns slowly. Each time they finish cooking, the fire is extinguished and relit only for cooking. If the groom is away on a journey, the bride will stop cooking with those pieces of wood until he returns. She would instead use another type of firewood. If the three big pieces of firewood are finished before the bride falls pregnant, she is sent back to her parents, an arrangement which is not communicated to her beforehand. It is assumed that the slow-burning logs will allow time enough for the woman to prove her fertility, failing which she is sent back home.

According to Wamwera tradition, a prospective wife should be from a family well known to her parents to avoid marrying into the same clan (*chipinga*), and she should be a respectable girl. Sometimes marriage could be arranged without the bride's knowledge. In such cases she could run away.

Comparing modern marriages with those of the past, one notes several differences. Marriages used to more permanent and stable. They were societal marriages because many members of the community took part and gave their blessings. These days, boys and girls marry without serious intent. Parents are hardly involved and where they are, making quick money from bridewealth is the main objective. They accept whoever comes to marry their daughters as long as he has money. Other considerations are generally secondary and are normally brushed aside. The groom no longer spends a night at the in-laws. Divorce rates are high. Sometimes a divorce takes place within a month of marriage. Custody of children, when divorce occurs, remains the concern of the wife and her relatives, namely her mother or grandmother. Conflicts related to marriage are reported to church elders more often than in the past. The social fabric that used to tie couples together is in many cases too weak or has disintegrated altogether.

Although marriages in the past were arranged by parents and maternal uncles who had the right to identify or endorse the girl to be married by the boy, such marriages were more permanent than present ones. Couples had more trust in each other than is the case today. At present boys and girls love and marry without the consent of their respective families. They marry easily and as easily divorce.

One of our informants is Mr. Iddi Maranga, a civil servant (cleaner) of 44 years of age. He remarks:

> I think these children are confused. They cheat each other. After a short while they leave each other, and the victim in most cases is the girl and her maternal relatives who have to take care of the offspring. There are almost no marriages these days as both parties are not serious about the institution. These days, boys and girls marry even when they cannot be self-reliant. A boy marries and expects his parents to take care of him and his wife. They do not engage in any economic activity, yet they get married. They seek no opinion from the clan or relatives. Marriage can take place anywhere, anytime, and with anybody. Most of such marriages do not last long—hardly a year.

Two of my daughters have children already. The eldest got pregnant at the age of 15 while in school. The culprit never married her. She is currently married to another man, but she has had two miscarriages. She does not have a child by her husband yet. I am taking care of her first child. My second daughter is now 18 years. She has two children. She had her first child at 15, after dropping out of school, and the second one at 18. She is not yet married. I am keeping and taking care of her and her children. There is no form of assistance from the boys who made her pregnant. The size of my family is beyond my financial capability. I have all these children to take care of and also grandchildren.

What about your own marriage and your children?

I got married in 1970 when I was 23 and my wife was 13 years old. My wife's first pregnancy occured at the age of 15. She had twins but one of them died. In total she had ten pregnancies, but eight children now survive. The other two died at a tender age. The doctor in charge of the district hospital here has also registered his concern about the size of my family and agreed to do a tubal ligation to my wife to prevent her from having more children. I am glad we did this, and it is now three years since we had our last child.

Iddi Maranga seems to feel the pinch of raising a large family under the present economic conditions, and he has displayed willingness to adopt modern family planning methods. Large families are no longer an ideal. An attitude change is slowly but surely taking place. However, while parents wish to limit the size of their own families, they have so far not succeeded in having such precautions taken by their children. Maybe in future, the numerous parents and maternal relatives who have taken care of grandchildren will accept the idea that their daughters and sons must have the means to prevent early pregnancies.

The secret of a lifelong marriage

Before we end this section we want to introduce Mrs. Chatanda Athumani, and her husband Mr. Athumani, 85, to the reader. They are both Wamwera and Muslims. We took the opportunity to talk with Mrs. Athumani as her husband had not yet returned home. She told us some of the facts about her life.

I went through the initiation when I was 14 to 15 years old. First of all, we were instructed how to behave and how to help ourselves and the elderly at the homestead. It was our duty to do the farming, fetch water, and cook. We were told not to be afraid if we liked a boy, but to listen to his needs. If we felt interested in him, we would end up with an agreement. Yes, we built temporary huts and tried to sleep in them. We pretended that we had a child, i.e., a log on my back was covered with cloth. We cooked food and we even ate together. The initiation, or to be precise, the seclusion period, lasted between three and six months—the time could vary. Occasionally, we were in mixed groups, girls and boys together.

Mrs. Athumani married when she was 22 years old, and her husband was 37. Her bridewealth was fifteen shillings. She gave birth to ten children. Only two sons are still alive, while all eight daughters died before the age of five. They fell ill and cried and cried without cease. The parents were not sure if it was malaria. The children's temperatures were very high and after a few days they died.

The sons married in the 1950s. The firstborn paid a bridewealth of twenty shillings, the second born 200 shillings. Now, the firstborn has divorced his first wife and married a new woman. The second born still has the same wife.

Why did the firstborn divorce? I did not get an immediate answer because Mr. Chetenye Athumani came home and took over the talking. He is a handsome man, tall and thin. He wears an worn beret. Like his wife, Mr. Athumani appears vital in spite of his great age. The spouses discussed the divorce of their firstborn son. Mr. Athumani then commented:

> During our lifetime we stuck together by using good sense. If one made mistakes, the other has been willing to forgive. We were not jealous like people are today. Our son immediately divorced his wife because she had made frequent mistakes with another man. Nowadays divorce is common. In our time everyone got married. Divorce was rare. Marriages lasted until one of the spouses died. I am worried about the children who are left without a father or mother. Grandparents care for many children.

How are your grandchildren today?

> My firstborn has six sons and two daughters. Both the daughters have husbands, but only one of the sons is married. The other five are still enjoying life in Dar es Salaam, Mtwara, and elsewhere. All the grandsons have travelled away, only the granddaughters remain here. My grandchildren were born at two year intervals beginning in 1965. So far our first son's second wife has no children.

> My second son has four daughters and two unmarried sons. Three of the daughters are married. One son is still small, the other has reached a marriageable age. He is about 20.

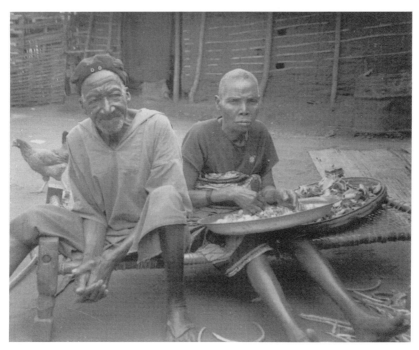

"Without good sense and indulgency   (Photo Rita Liljeström)
marriage does not work".

Looking at the old spouses, one senses the mutual understanding and coordination that has evolved over six decades. Still strong, they are troubled by their grandsons who "enjoy life" in distant places, and their firstborn who has divorced the mother of his eight children.

How did they succeed in staying together? The answer is simple, according to Mr. Athumani. What is demanded is good sense and indulgence. Without these two, marriage does not work. You have to be able to do your part for the family, and you have to overlook the occasional weakness of the other.

Victims of custom and change

Our original point of departure was the reproductive risks that teenage girls face: the unwanted pregnancies, expulsion from school, single motherhood, frequent anaemia, complications in pregnancy, not to mention maternal and infant mortality. While our initial studies focused on the girls, we soon became aware that they are but an integral part of a larger whole. Therefore, we expanded our approach to include changes in ethnic marriages and family patterns and in the pool of girls' boyfriends.

Victims of early motherhood

I paid a visit to the local mission hospital and the hospital gynaecologist, a German Catholic nun known to be devoted to her work. She was willing to assist me, but the data they have for young girls are not categorized by tribes. Available records at the hospital do show that teenage pregnant girls regularly visit the MCH (Mother and Child Health) clinic. Three out of five women who come for check-ups are teenage girls. Some of these may be in their second or third pregnancies. The record also shows that almost 50 per cent of teenagers who deliver at the hospital experience complications, including infant deaths, maternal deaths, and severe (but rare) cases caused of vaginal or rectal rupture during delivery. The doctor told of severe rupture cases and I was able to talk to these girls.

At first, the girls indicated that they were married. However, further probing revealed that they were in fact cohabiting with the men who were responsible for their pregnancies: "The man is my child's father, so I decided to identify myself with him." It is worth noting the phrase "to identify myself with him", not "to marry him." They all seemed convinced that the men were unwilling to marry them. The men enjoyed having sex, but were unprepared to shoulder the obligations that arose from that enjoyment. Besides, the girls' medical condition probably frightened them. One of the girls lamented that:

> ... my parents forced me into marriage when I was 15 years old and still in school. I had to leave school and marry a man unknown to me. He was 20 years old. But after I got into this state, neither my husband nor my parents have ever assisted me. They came to see me at the hospital during the first few weeks. After seeing my miserable condition, they gave up. They never came anymore. They abandoned me until I could get cured. I underwent five operations. It was only then that they came to see me. I am now working at the hospital and one of my duties is to counsel other girls who have fallen victims to severe ruptures.

Bahati, another victim, was still in bed during my visit. She had been transferred from another mission hospital where she had been operated on twice without success. Bahati looked pale and innocent, not aware of her fate. She, however, was in pain and was bothered by the temporary opening in her abdomen through which urine and faeces were being drained into a plastic bag. She has to empty the bag often, as she has no control over her functions. Bahati complained of loneliness because only Maria, an earlier victim of rupture, and hospital personnel came and talked to her. She lamented: "No relatives come to see me. Not even the boy who made me pregnant."

A visit to the children's ward gave me an opportunity to talk to four teenage mothers whose children were admitted to the hospital. The children, aged between two weeks and one year looked sick and weak. They suffered from diseases such as malaria, diarrhoea, and anaemia. Only Mama Kami was married. Hers was neither a customary nor a religious marriage, but a civil one. Her husband visited her occasionally, but mostly her maternal relatives came to see her. The other three mothers did not want to talk about the fathers of their children. Salima, whose child was one year old, complained: "Once I delivered this baby, the man was nowhere to be seen and he has never seen the baby. He decided to move out of our village and I have no idea of his whereabouts."

All the young mothers indicated that they received support from maternal relatives. They all admitted that they would prefer to get married because it is easier to meet the vagaries of life when two people live together than alone, but they wished to marry a man other than the fathers of their firstborn children, the men who had let them down.

Left on their own

Mr. Muhammed Chitindi, is 80 years old and his wife 70 years old. They have spent all their life in the village, which means that they moved with the village when it was relocated three miles to its present place. This was when the *ujamaa* villages were established.

We inquired about their early family relationships and the old man had ready answers to questions, which he clearly expected. Obviously, the news about what we were interested in had spread like wildfire through the village. His initiation into malehood included instructions about farming, building of houses, and storage facilities. He was trained and worked as blacksmith for twenty years.

When Mr. Chitindi married in 1937, he paid forty shillings. He was then 25 years old. The bride was chosen by his father. She was 15

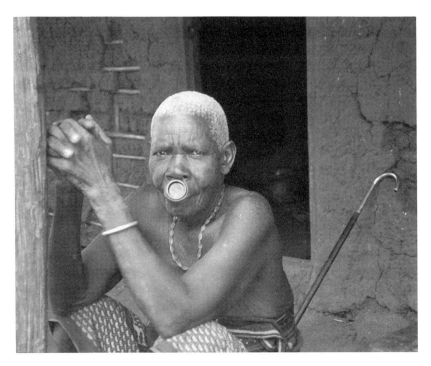

When slave hunters captured people for slave trade,   (Photo Rita Liljeström)
young women had plugs inserted into their upper
jaw-bone, between the nose and lip. This was a way
to escape being taken by Arabs for slavery.

years old. They still live together. She bore him a son and three daughters. Now the old couple have twelve grandchildren. The maternal uncle, i.e., the wife's brother, lives twenty-five kilometres from Ruangwa. "My wife moved to my homestead", Mr. Chitindi says.

At first I felt embarrassed by Mr. Chitindi's wife; she had a round black plug inserted into her upper lip. It is made from the *makonde* tree. Mr. Chitindi explained this mutilation of his wife. In the past, when slave hunters captured people for the slave trade, young women had these plugs inserted into their upper jaw-bone, between the nose and the lip. This was a way to escape being taken by Arabs for slavery. They left those girls whose faces made them too horrifying to be taken with the slave convoys. When this old woman was a bride of 15, the plug must have tortured her. By this time, the wooden piece has sunk into the flesh and stopped causing pain.

Mr. Chitindi told us about his children.

> All my children are married and live with their partners. My son was initiated when he was 10 years old. He married at 18. His bridewealth was 4,000 shillings. My daughters were initiated when they were between 9 and 12 years old. Their age of marriage varied between 17 and 20. The bridewealth I received when I married off my oldest daughter was 2,500 shillings while I got 9,000 for the youngest. The bridewealth for my middle daughter fell between those sums. It is good for a girl to be married, and easy for a boy to marry.

> All our children selected their spouses on their own. We parents participated in the weddings. Today, all the children live far away from Ruangwa. We are old and need someone to look after us, but our daughters are in the hands of their husbands. And when it comes to helping relatives, even sisters are nowadays under their husbands control.

What does it look like if you compare how things were when you were young with how they are for your grandson? What remains the same, what has changed?

> In the past we lived in family groups consisting of three generations. It was easy for the old men and women to control everything in the community. The *ujamaa* villages broke apart family groups. Boys and girls started to look for jobs elsewhere and travelled away. The system of homesteads has broken down.

While others have spoken about clan disruption and loss of Wamwera customs, Mr. Chitindi bears witness to the broken homesteads and the abandonment of an old couple. There is nobody to look after their needs.

A lost daughter?

An educated and retired Mwera teacher, Lucas Mbina, narrates his experience of the contradictions between tradition and modernization as follows :

> I went to school with the maternal uncle of my wife-to-be. We became friends and used to talk about his sister's daughter. I became interested and decided to spend one of my holidays at his place so that I could meet his niece. After seeing her, I went to my maternal uncle and elder brother to tell them of my interests. They agreed to initiate an engagement. By then, I had completed schooling and started teaching.

After engagement, *kulomba,* I lived with my in-laws and my marriage was arranged. My maternal uncles and brothers paid bridewealth. The marriage took place in a Catholic church. I was 26 years old while my bride was 19. I lived with my in-laws shortly before being transferred to work outside the locality. The first child was born in the same year. My wife had eleven pregnancies altogether. Four babies were lost; two were miscarriages and two died of sickness. We have, therefore, been blessed with seven children, four girls and three boys. All of them are grown up, independent, and working.

Of my four girls, two have children out-of-wedlock. One daughter is married to a white man and lives with him in Germany. She is a nurse by profession and worked in a church hospital. The white man was a secondary school teacher in our area. They met and became friends. It took them a long time to inform us. We always thought they were mere friends and nothing serious would come out of their relationship. Never had we thought of our child marrying a white man. When they broke the news to us, we were shocked and tried to prevent it from happening. We knew we had lost a daughter, and more so, we were concerned about society's attitude to her. How would she merge our tradition and his?

However, with no concern for those worries, our daughter went ahead and arranged her church marriage to the white man. As you can see on that wedding photo on the wall, my daughter got married to a white man. They currently live in Germany. They visit us once in awhile. However, both my wife and I are extremely concerned as she has no children. I don't know what the meaning is. Will she ever have children? I have heard that some white people marry and prefer not to have children. If this is the case, why? After all, they are rich! As for their marriage there were no traditions attached to it because the groom was not a Mwera. We wanted to be fair to our son-in-law. The marriage was purely a Christian one. We could not even demand bridewealth as it was a marriage we were not happy with. Things were beyond our control.

"We wanted to be fair to our son-in-law", as Lucas Mbina puts it when referring to the white man who had married his daughter, reflects a point of departure—call it social tolerance, understanding, or accommodation. This always occurs in the acculturation process. But while the Mbinas are willing to let matters stand, they appear to be constantly haunted by the idea that "we have lost her", an idea well rooted in the sociocultural practices that tie an individual to her clan and ethnic group. For a girl to be married to a man and be taken out of the community is regarded as "losing her". And yet Mbina does not seem to show such concern about his two daughters working in the "towns outside their community". Why does he not regard these

There is no question that the Mbinas are caught up in the contradictions of modernization. They must learn to live with them as the reality of the day. Change has to come, because interaction and exposure will always make it possible.

The erosion of the matrilineal order of the Wamwera

This study has indicated some shifting trends and practices in marriage among the Wamwera. As early as 1930s the Wamwera matriliny began to change to patriliny. It has since been replaced by married couples living by themselves or with the parents of the groom. There are fewer and fewer arranged marriages. Youth make their own choice of spouses, decisions that are encouraged by a sense of freedom. These trends imply that the current generation is breaking away from the old customs related to marriage. However, there are still intermarriages involving a mixture of practices that sometimes lead to an increased rate of divorce. However, increased rates of divorce and intermarriage among ethnic groups are seemingly a reflection of freedom of choice. Indeed, there are young men who choose not to marry while still conceiving children. The young generation is rebelling against mutual dependency and control. People are disengaged from the common interest of the clan. The current realities are complex.

Extended families are breaking up and are being replaced by nuclear families. The reality is that matriliny cannot be sustained. Forces of change are too much for it. Bridewealth is no longer paid to the maternal uncle unless he has been responsible for the upbringing of his niece. The parents are assuming this role exclusively.

This study also reveals another important fact: each system of marriage has its own inner logic. A change to a critical part of the system threatens the very system itself. The erosion of old norms, customs, and traditions among the Wamwera is inevitable. It has come and will continue to take its course. The issue, therefore, is not to worry about past Wamwera customs but about how to replace them. A vacuum means lack of direction, and this is apparently the case. Parents are becoming rather lax about their parental responsibilities. The men are taking advantage of the transition of obligations from uncle to father. The women generate income from sexual services. The traditionalists blame the young generation while the young generation blame the old ones for conservatism and fear of change. Actually, it is not solely a question of age and generation, but much generation blame the old ones for conservatism and fear of change. Actually, it is not solely a question of age and generation, but much more one of gender, namely the diverse and sometimes incompatible interests of men and women.

References

Abdallah, Yohanna B., 1949, *The Yaos; Their Customs and Manners*. Ed. and transl. by Meredith Sanderson.

Alpers, E.A., 1965, "Towards a History of Expansion of Islam in East Africa: the Matrilineal Peoples of the Southern Interior", in Rangers, T.O. and I. Kimambo (eds.), *Historical Survey of African Religion*.

Ayisi, E.O, 1972, *Introduction to Study of African Culture*. London: Heinemann.

Beidelman, T.O., 1970, *The Kaguru, A matrilineal people of East Africa*. New York: Holt, Reinehart and Winston.

Hokororo, M., 1961. *The influence of church on local customs at Lukuledi*. Ndanda: Mission Press.

Ingham, K., 1965, *A history of East Africa*. London: Longmans.

Kamazima, A., 1994, *The Girl Child in Tunduru District*. UNICEF report.

Lamburn, R.G.P., 1950, *Yao Customs and Manners*. Tanganyika Notes and Records.

Mair, Lucy, 1974, *African Societies*. London: Cambridge University Press.

Mitchell, J.C., 1959, "The Yao of Nyasaland", in E. Colson and M. Gluckman (eds.), *Seven Tribes of British Central Africa*. Manchester University Press.

—1956, *The Yao Village*. Report of an Ethnological Expedition. Manchester University Press.

Seligman, C.O., 1939, *Races of Africa*. London: Thornton Butterworth Ltd.

Shuma, Mary, 1994, "The Case of Matrilineal Mwera of Lindi", in *Chelewa, Chelewa. The Dilemma of Teenage Girls*. Uppsala: Scandinavian Institute of African Studies.

Wagi-Rubereeza, V., 1994, *Ten Makonde Folk Tales*.

—1993, *Images of Women in Makonde Folk Tales*. A Status Report.

Chapter 4
Training by Symbolism and Imagery
—The Case of Wagogo and Wayao

Zubeida Tumbo-Masabo

After exploring the increased role of mothers in teaching their daughters about sexuality and reproductive health in urban areas (Tumbo-
Masabo, 1994), I wanted to investigate the situation in rural areas
among the Wayao and Wagogo. These are peoples with different lineage systems, i.e., matrilineal versus patrilineal. I wished to see
whether there would be the same differences observed by Ntukula
(1994:113) namely, that initiation ceremonies are still an important
stage in defining womanhood in the matrilineal societies of Wamwera, Wayao, and Waluguru and that these rites are elaborate, but the
situation is different in the patrilineal communities she visited among
the Wangoni of Peramiho and Maposeni, where the initiation ceremonies are withering away. Thus, I was interested to establish whether these were isolated cases of a difference in the two types of lineage
concerning the importance of initiation rites or a general phenomenon. Another objective of my study was to examine the differences
and similarities in the way information on sexuality and reproduction
is disseminated from one generation to the next with the aim of seeing
how such information affected teenage motherhood in the research
areas.

The study was undertaken among two communities in Tanzania.
One was the Wagogo of Simba Chinzachi (also pronounced as Simba
Kinzaki) in Dodoma rural district, about twenty kilometres southwest
of the famous educational and health centre of Mundemu, which is a
few kilometres off the Dodoma–Arusha road. The other community is
the Wayao of Mbesa village in Nalasi ward, Tunduru district, about
twenty kilometres south of Tunduru town. Mbesa is a long established education and health centre run by missionaries but with a sizeable
Muslim population. Both villages depend on agriculture for their
economy. The main crops in Mbesa are cashew as a cash crop, sorg-

hum (*mtama*), cassava, pigeon peas as food crops and maize, which is both food and cash crop. In Simba Chinzachi the main food crops are peanuts, hard nuts (*njugumawe*), bullrush millet (*uwele*), and maize, which is used as both food and cash crop.

At first I intended to use only one-to-one interviews, but I had to use other methodologies to adduce information from less willing respondents. The most productive method was focus group discussions, especially in determining the matrimonial changes among Wayao, general cultural issues, and changes in behaviour and expectations of parents and children.

I had four focus group discussions, two in each research area: one with men (estimated age 55 and above) and another with women (estimated age 50 and above). Most people are not sure how old they are. A woman who looked much older than myself, whom I greeted with "*shikamoo*", told me she was 30 years old.

I had a total of nine respondents in the one-to-one interviews among Wayao, six teenage mothers and three of their mothers, and twelve respondents among Wagogo, six teenage mothers, four of their mothers, one aunt and one *ngariba* (initiator and circumciser) who was also a trained traditional birth attendant. However, most of the respondents did not wish to respond to my questions dealing with the content of initiation training, which seemed to be the major means of teaching girls about reproduction and family life. Parents could teach their children good manners and discipline only. They were not expected to touch on the information which was imparted during initiations, For example, among Wayao, mothers are not supposed to tell their girls anything about their bodies. That is done during the first initiation (*msondo*), which takes place very early in puberty, i.e., around the age of 9 or 10, and at subsequent initiations.

Respondents were not forthcoming because of the strict oaths taken during initiation. Indeed, they would be punished even prior to taking the oath. The *manyakanga* (trainers) and *mangariba* (circumcisers) go through a rigorous oath-taking procedure to ensure that they do divulge the secrets of the training. Hence, all my attempts to get a trainer to tell me even a little about what goes on failed completely among the Wayao and I could only obtain anecdotal information from one Wagogo *ngariba*. Also, I learned that in order to be a trainer, one needs to be able to protect oneself and the novices against witchcraft. The trainer goes through many of processes and much oath taking to secure such protective powers. In most oaths, the takers are warned against the misfortune that will befall them if they reveal information. Therefore, most respondents gave me the standard answer that I received in my pilot study, namely that girls receive training in hygiene and good manners and nothing else during the initiation. However, one Wayao teenage mother was extremely cooperative. She was from the house that I stayed in and her father was my contact in the village. It seemed that I had already created enough rapport with the family to win her confidence. However, she was not sure of the wording of the songs used at the initiations she had gone through. Nonetheless, she was able to provide me with the broad wording and meaning of some of the common songs.

Initiation songs call not only for knowledge of everyday use of language, but its euphemisms, symbolic meanings, and imagery which are not easy for a young person to grasp, even after completing the first or even second round of initiation. This also true for a newcomer to a language, who is in the area for a one or two month fieldtrip. Moreover, when I saw the numerous corrections done on Cory's (1951a&b)[1] collections, probably by mother-tongue speakers of languages in the collections, it made me think that any rushed collection would end up similarly flawed.

The life of a Myao Girl

What has the older generation to say?

The focus group discussions I had among Wayao opened my eyes to a number of things that I had taken for granted in my pilot study. For example, in whose compound does the family live? Is it the wife's clan's land or the husband's compound, i.e., matrilocal or patrilocal? This is important in determining who makes the final decision on the different issues pertaining to the upbringing of children and planning different ceremonies that accompany initiation rites. The Yao put much emphasis on the initiation of girls and boys, especially if both parents are Yao.

---

[1] Hans Cory was a British government administrator in the then Tanganyika. He was appointed government sociologist in 1943. He was interested in and knowledgeable about African songs and dances, tribal ceremonies, and customary law. He has made numerous collections about different ethnic groups in the abovementioned fields. The collections can be found at the University of Dar es Salaam and the Tanzania National Archives.

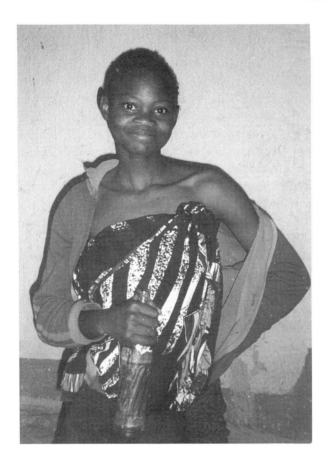

A Myao girl
(Photo Rita Liljeström)

If the parents live in the wife's family compound, then the uncle, usually the eldest brother of the wife, will be the final decisionmaker. If they live in the husband's compound, then the father will agree with his wife as to what is best for their children, but the uncle must be informed of their decision, though he cannot usually reverse it. However, a child can conspire with the uncle to have decisions reconsidered when these are not in his/her favour and the uncle can try to convince the parents on his/her behalf.

Who takes care of the child? Sometimes an uncle can ask to raise a sister's child, and such request usually goes undebated, because in Yao custom the uncle is senior to the father. However, a lot of care is taken in cases of intermarriage. The types of initiation ceremonies that parents go through determine the initiation ceremonies that the child goes through.

Sometimes, children born of mothers of another ethnic group are not initiated according to Yao customs. This is because the children have to go through similar initiation rites to their parents, for fear that children will be disrespectful if they believe that they know things that their parents do not know. This response was especially common regarding the type of education children obtain in modern schools. People in the discussion groups felt that children who go through the school system are spoiled and do not adhere to society's norms, hence the increase in the out-of-wedlock pregnancy.

Another factor that emerged was the need for continuous peer training of children in family life (*jinsi ya kuishi na watu*). Most of the people in the discussion groups felt that the old training system through initiation rites, that required everyone who had attended an initiation rite to participate on a continuous basis in similar initiations, was of immense help in keeping and expanding the knowledge gained during initiation. It is impossible to do this nowadays, as people are mobile and children have to attend school, sometimes far away. Most of the training during the initiation is done by peers who have gone through the initiation in the previous intake under close supervision of *manyakanga*, in the case of girls, and *makungwi*, in the case of boys.

The most important thing I learned from the focus group discussions was that people were prepared to view me as a willing novice, while during my initial contact through the pilot study, they tended to treat me as an intruder.

Findings from individual interviews

I had very limited responses concerning initiation in the individual interviews, but I was prepared for this. From the only grandmother that I interviewed during the main study, I learned that I could not be initiated as I had been told in the pilot study. I was told that the earlier remark was only a joke: the Ngoni (my ethnic group) and the Yao have a joking relationship (*utani*). In a joking relationship, which can be intergenerational (see Jacobson-Widding, 1984) or more commonly in Tanzania, between ethnic groups (see Lucas and Tengo, 1975), one can fib, obfuscate or even exchange obscenities without provoking anger in the other party. Moreover, since I come from a different ethnic group, I could not be initiated through Yao customs, unless I was given my baby-name by a Myao, i.e., had a Myao as a *somo*. To the Yao, a *somo* is a "friend", someone who names one after him or herself when one is born. Such relationship commands great respect among the Yao. Usually, contact is kept with *somos* and they contribute much to bringing up a child.

However, the interviewee was not willing to give me any new information besides what she thought I new from initiation in my own ethnic group. She would only tell me what they are taught about hygiene during initiation, because she knows that the Ngoni are taught about keeping clean and how to take care of the menstrual cloth (*mpati*) at home and away from home, great emphasis being put on guarding against bad bodily odours (including one's clothing), which are taken to be a sign of uncleanliness (see also Ntukula, 1994:106).

The most useful information came from one teenage mother who was willing to tell me and even demonstrate to me the different actions (*vitendo*) that are taught in the three initiation ceremonies:

Msondo, which is done when a girl is 8 to 9 years old, just at the onset of puberty. Here she is taught about self-respect and respect for parents and other elders; cooking (which training continues after the ceremony); cleanliness of the environment, the utensils she uses, and her own body; *ngoma* playing and especially wiggling the waist. *Msondo* takes seven or eight nights. Most of the teaching is done at night.

This type of initiation is performed under cashew trees which are usually found near the house used for the initiation. The initiation is generally done to a group of girls under the guidance of a *nyakanga*. The *nyakanga* is helped by *warindembo* (pubescent girls who have not had their menarche but have themselves gone through *msondo*). Day-by-day activities are as follows:

Day 1.   The novices are secluded and offerings are made to propitiate the spirits of the dead (*tambiko*) for the safety of the novices during the initiation. They are daubed with flour (*mbopezi*) and a leader of novices is chosen by the *nyakanga*. No definite criteria were given for the choice, but usually one who is known to be disciplined is preferred.

Ngoma is played overnight and the novices are supposed to stay awake throughout the night and they are bathed by rolling (*kugaagaa*) in *ndembo kayoga* (cold water mixed with powder from herbs). A song during this episode is known as "*Mchenyendela mkanileje pano*" (a person who cuts/cultivates a border carefully resides here)—the theme being: Look before you leap. The aim of the song is to teach the novice to be patient and cautious.

Day 2. The novices sleep during the day and wake around 2:00 to 3:00 pm and dance until late in the evening.

Day 3. The novices bath again by rolling and then *mwari ndembo* (the novice's escort) dances. This involves wiggling the waist under a winnowing basket *(ungo)*. The song on this occasion is *"Nyanyamila kali munyumba"* (one who tiptoes in the house). A thief or a person who wants to eavesdrop usually tiptoes so as to escape attention. The aim of the song is to warn girls against being thieves and liars.

Day 4. The novices dance half the night until midnight.

Day 5. More difficult tasks are introduced. The novices are required to use their mouths to pick up six or seven strung beads which are laid horizontally on the floor. The novice is supposed to move with her legs wide apart and bend her head to reach for the beads by mouth and give them to the *nyakanga*, who sits at the end of the line. The aim of the action is to teach the girl to restrain herself instead of revealing everything she sees or knows and to conceal the wrongdoings of her parents and other elders, and not to go into rooms without notifying the occupants *(kupiga hodi)*.

Day 6. The novices fast and they are kept indoors while *mwari ndembo* (the escorts) sit in the backyard of the house. The *nyakanga*, with the help of female elders, draws on the ground many stars, a moon, and an old man with a hydrocele *(mshipa)*. The drawing made with millet fluor is done while the escorts are blindfolded.

The stars and the moon teach initiates about nature and the belief that the hydrocele comes from being uncleanly. Cleanliness here means both the body and of the heart; one should care for ones parents and be kind to other people.

During the evening, the novices are given *msondoka*, a bitter medicine made from the *msondoka plant*, to make them vomit.

The novice is supposed to vomit the childhood milk, marking the end of childhood and entry into girlhood.

Day 7.   The novices are taken to bathe in the river and their heads are shaven. They are then taken from another house, not the one they were secluded in. Each novice is given a new name for girlhood, and is never again to be called by her childhood name.Novices are then seated in the frontyard to receive presents from parents and well wishers.

During these seven days, the undisciplined novice can face severe punishment, such as skipping on one leg with one arm high in the air. If she cries, she is given a pot to fill with tears. Or she can be beaten three or four times with a thorny *msondoka* branch, or be told to crawl on her knees to fetch her mother who is hidden under a bed, where the novice is not supposed to look. The paternal aunt can help the novice by paying a specified amount of money as a fine.

The mother of a novice is not expected to teach the girl anything other than what she has been taught at the *msondo*.

Unyago wa kuvunja ungo—initiation at menarche

This initiation is also known as *chiguluka kiziza* (to step over the cooking place/stove). For the first seven days, when the novice is still menstruating, she is left to rest and eat well. At this time, she is taught about bodily hygiene, how to keep herself clean and concealed during menstruation, and show respect for elders and her future husband.

The novice goes through a whole day's training on the eighth day, when she is also supposed to fast. She eats in the evening after the teaching.

An *msondoka* plant is found and a hole is dug around the roots. The trainer *(kungwi)* sits behind the novice and an elderly woman removes the novice's pubic hair with warm ashes. After that, three seeds, white, black, and red, are brought and the following meanings are attached to the seeds: the white seed denotes the genital discharges *(utoko)* the girl has been seeing since childhood, black denotes menarche blood or the first days of menstruation, and red denotes continuing menstrual blood. The novices are also taught that they have to abstain from sex as soon as they reach menopause and that they should also not have sex during menstruation.

Much symbolism is attached to the sexual act. For example, one is not supposed to remove the feathers of a chicken in front of elders as this is associated with the removal of pubic hair, which has to be done in strict privacy.

The girl is also taught how to keep herself clean during menstruation by using a piece of cloth (*mpati*). She is told that if she is at home she must dry the menstrual cloth under her mattress or in between a folded mat, but not at the head-rest. If one is travelling, the *mpati* is dried by being hung from a string tied around the waist.

The girl is then given strung beads of three colours: white, black, and red. She uses the beads when she gets married to communicate to her husband about her menstrual cycle. The white beads shows that she is not having her period, the black beads denotes that she has started her period, and she uses the red beads to show that she is in the middle of her period. She puts the beads under her husband's pillow. Boys are taught about the beads during their initiation.

The three colours, black, white, and red are also used as a ritual symbols in other societies, especially in the lower Congo (Jacobson-Widding, 1979). The red is associated with procreation, fatherhood, and power to defend against evil spirits (p. 286). Black is associated with being healthy (pp. 181–3). However, my respondent did not associate the colours with any other beliefs besides showing the different stages of the menstrual cycle.

After the second initiation, the mother and other older female relatives who live with the girl are supposed to train her in cooking and good housekeeping and prepare her for her future life as a housewife. She is constantly reminded of her destiny by words such as, "*Ndio utakuwa unafanya hivyo ukiwa na mumeo?*" (Is that what you are going to do when you are with your husband?)

After this, the girl is expected to marry once she has been through another year of attending initiations, this time as an escorting novice (*mwari ndembo*). This means she will marry when she is between 16 and 17 years of age. Usually, the birth of the first child occurs within a year or two of marriage, making teenage motherhood a normal exigency for Myao woman.

Unyago wa uzazi—initiation at childbirth

At this time, the woman is accompanied by her husband and they are both taught how to care for their coming child. They are taught about labour and where the baby will come from. The husband may be exempted if he has gone through similar training in the case of a serial or polygamous marriage. They are also taught how to cut the umbilical cord and how to remove the placenta, should this be necessarily. The husband is taught these things so that he can assist his wife if they cannot get help from a female relative. A lot of suspicion is attached to help being sought outside the family, as most people believe that the first birth is crucial in assuring safe subsequent births.

Many symbols are used in the training to get the information across. Simple items are used, such as pots (which symbolize the uterus and the vagina), a banana (symbolizing the penis), and flour (the reddish millet flour which symbolizes the bleeding during labour. At the initiation, the pregnant woman and her husband are taught about the signs of labour, such as the breaking of the waters. For this, the millet flour and water are used as symbols. They are taught that the baby will come through the vagina, where the husband has been inserting his penis. This is demonstrated by using a pot and a banana. They are told that the baby comes head first but they should also be ready for other types of arrival, such as breech births. However, they are told to seek help early and that the husband should only help his wife in cases of emergency. Otherwise, as soon as the signs of labour occur, he should call for assistance from family members, who usually live nearby. Generally, a young wife lives near her mother's compound.

This initiation is usually done during late pregnancy. At this stage, the woman is supposed not to have sex until her child is walking. Hence, after the initiation, the woman is given a black cloth (*knack*) to tie under her loins and across her back (*kupiga winda*). She uses the black cloth to massage the baby's limbs until the baby can walk, so that the baby stays strong. A similar procedure is used as therapy for fever and burns among the Manyika of Zimbabwe (Jacobson-Widding, 1989), where a mother puts a piece of cloth between her legs in the evening in order to collect vaginal fluid to cool the baby's fever or burns.

Moreover, the Myao woman is taught that men are monsters when it comes to sexual desire and it is up to the woman to safeguard herself. A song to this effect is known as *"wangalicha naza kutomba"* (you should not have lain on me). It is a song about a woman who laments to her husband that they should not have had sex.

The childbirth rite concludes the rites of passage that a Myao woman goes through.

The life of a Mgogo Girl

The focus group discussion

The focus group discussions with Wagogo elders were valuable in teaching me that the tradition of female circumcision is important to them. Wagogo believe that girls who are not circumcised are susceptible to *lawalawa*, which seems to be a genital fungal disease. They believe this can cause death if it is not attended to, either through circumcision or by means of intense hospital care, which is unavailable in most areas. All the participants were aware that the government is against circumcision of girls but most did not agree with the government's view that female circumcision leads to difficult or even dangerous births and an increase in maternal mortality. Most of the women thought, that the restriction was advocated by educated women (*wasomi*) who did not appreciate other people's customs. They gave me examples of women who had given birth to many children safely and commented that many maternal deaths occur among uncircumcised women. One of them lamented that the government takes no action in trying to prevent *lawalawa* but hinders people who are trying to defend themselves against this killer disease.

It should be noted that most literature on female circumcision aims at finding ways to ban it (MacLean and Graham, 1983; Slack, 1988; *WIN News*, 1993; Walker, 1993; Toubia, 1994) and most of the women I talked to know of the campaigns but do not agree with them. According to most of these women, the training offered during circumcision on how to live with people outside one's family, and the friendship and comradeship fostered at that time are more important than the circumcision itself. And nobody agreed with the argument that female circumcision diminishes a woman's sexual pleasure and it is a way for men to control women's sexuality. Most of them said that female circumcision dried the female genitalia and made sexual intercourse more pleasurable for both partners because wet sex is messy and smelly, and therefore less pleasurable.

However, I also learned that girls are sent for circumcision much earlier than was the case before, due to the fact that children have to attend school and parents would like the girls circumcised before they are polluted by the modern world. Now girls as young as 8 are circumcised, as against 12 or 13 traditionally. However, during circumcision, girls are not taught anything about menarche, reproduction, or sexuality, but are taught to respect their elders, to keep secrets, and not to speak about things they see or hear unless they are called upon to do so by those concerned.

The most important initiation rite among Wagogo is *jando*. *Jando* combines initiation rites and circumcision. It is held for both boys and girls. They use similar names for people who are involved in the initiation and circumcision, e.g., the circumcisers are called *ngariba* for both sexes and the trainers are called *nyakanga*. The incision of the clitoris is compared to the incision of the prepuce, i.e., circumcision gets rid of menacing outgrowths.

Most women who participated in the focus group discussion held that government does not respect people's traditions and that independence has not changed the disregard for traditional culture that characterized government in the colonial era. Though I tried to explain that the incision of the clitoris had a negative effect on the health of women, especially in childbirth, almost all of them did not believe me. This argument lost credibility because with deterioration of health services, the occurrence of maternal death is widespread even among uncircumcised women.

Training and life at initiation

The teaching of tribal traditions, behaviour, and morals is not explicit and the instruction is usually through songs. However, complete understanding of the songs may only be acquired later by attending other novices' initiations (see also Cory, 1951a and 1951b). Also, words are given different unusual meanings (*mizimu*) and novices who cannot repeat them accurately are punished. Sometimes punishment is given for no apparent cause but just to instil strict obedience towards seniors.

In earlier times, girls were circumcised in groups of no less than five and the circumciser and trainer were paid in kind, in the form of a goat, flour etc. Nowadays, with the cash economy, they are paid in cash, usually the equivalent of the price of a goat. Consequently, the ceremonies are now more costly and families have to pool resources before they can send their children for circumcision. Circumcision is performed during the cold season to hasten healing.

On the day of circumcision, which is usually during the full moon, the girls are taken far from home and there is much singing and drumming by the older women who escort the girls. The noises are made to muffle the screaming of the girls. Even though they are warned against screaming during circumcision, the girls told me the procedure was too painful for silence. The songs that are sung at this time are to instil independence in the girls, that they should not rely on their parents so much as they are about to leave their families and live with outsiders, be it husbands or in-laws, who might not be as supportive as their own kin. The girls are also taught about the virtues of diligence, perseverance, and kindness.

The girls can stay up to three months in seclusion after circumcision if they have finished school, which is rare nowadays. Most of them stay for one month only. At this time, they are under the care of peers who have already undergone circumcision. These peers help the circumcized girls not to hurt themselves by holding their legs apart until they heal. They also make sure that the genital apertures are not covered during healing. In earlier days, circumcision coincided with menarche, but with the pressure of schooling and especially the movement to boarding schools, parents send their girls for circumcision at a much earlier age. The peers, who are considered as *madada* (sisters), act as private tutors to novices and teach them *mizimu* (hidden meaning of words used in initiation) and songs. The peers and novices develop permanent friendships and usually the peers become advisors to the girls on family life matters, sometimes on a long-term basis.

The next initiation is after menarche, when a girl is initiated individually by her aunts and other elderly women relatives. During this initiation, the girl is taught how to take care of her sanitary cloths and especially how to wash them and dry them discreetly. Most of the respondents observed that nowadays girls are not as careful as they used to be. Nowadays, the superstitions that were attached to non-concealment of sanitary cloths are disregarded as primitive by girls who have gone to school. But the older generation still believes that fertility can be harmed if an evil person gets hold of one's sanitary cloth.

Though infertility is not considered cause for divorce among Wagogo (see also Cory, 1957), it can lead to a man marrying other wives and neglecting his infertile wife. Impotence is a valid cause for a woman to leave her husband. Therefore, men are eager to prove their potency as early as possible, while women seem to have a similar urge to have babies at a very young age to prove their fertility.

The last initiation rite is performed about a week before marriage. The wife-to-be is put in seclusion for a week and she is trained by her aunts and other elderly women relatives (*mabibi*), sometimes with the help of a *nyakanga*, for her new life as a wife. During this time she is told to respect her husband and her in-laws and all her new family. Marriage problems are to be solved within the framework of her new family and she should not come rushing home to her mother and father. The teachings of diligence, perseverance, and kindness are re-iterated. One of the respondents told me that in earlier days *jando* (circumcision) coincided with marriage and hence there was no need to repeat the training as is the case nowadays.

Conclusion

Initiation is given high priority among the Wayao and Wagogo. In fact, parents who cannot send their children for initiation are despised and the uninitiated are called names and are not regarded as grown-ups, even if they are elderly. Therefore, initiation is an important rite of passage into adulthood in both these societies. Parents are ready to sacrifice what little they have, to seek assistance from relatives, and even take on loans to initiate their children.

It is also evident from the study that Wayao and Wagogo depend on the teaching of traditional trainers during the different stages of initiation, and that many beliefs are attached to the whole process of initiation. Though parents, especially mothers, shape the lives of their children during childhood, most of the teaching after that is left to the initiators. The parents are only there to affirm what has been taught during the initiation and they cannot teach anything new until the next stage of initiation.

In this regard, repeated teenage pregnancies are not the result of mother-daughter communication but may be influenced by the teaching that is given to the girls during initiation. There is no time in the initiation when one is taught that falling pregnant when young is wrong, though girls are warned against pregnancy out-of-wedlock, especially if they are still in school. Among the Wagogo, sexual inter-course before circumcision is taboo, while Yao girls are punished severely if it is known that they have engaged in sexual intercourse before puberty. Hence initiations set the time for different activities in a woman's lifecycle and prepare women psychologically for them. Some of the activities that demarcate womanhood are sexual intercourse in marriage and procreation.

Among rural Wagogo, it is almost impossible for an uncircumcised man or woman to get married. It is only among urbanized Wagogo that circumcision is dying. All the Wagogo women I interviewed held that an uncircumcised woman stinks, especially Wagogo women (maybe they did not want to offend me as they knew, that I was not circumcised) and that they become susceptible to *lawalawa*. Therefore, government should try to provide effective health and sanitation services to address those concerns rather than apply legal sanctions which people will attempt to circumvent.

Another observation I made is that most of the girls marry as soon as they finish primary education, while boys stood more chance of obtaining further education. Parents would find means to give boys further education by sending them to relatives in urban areas, while girls would be married off as soon as they finished primary school, especially if they are not selected for admission to government secondary schools. Such circumstances force girls to marry early, as there is no other prospect for them and they cannot wait until 18, the age which the government believes to be right for marriage and childbirth. Early marriage and childbirth become not only normal for girls but are the response to an unaddressed predicament.

References

Cory, H., 1951a, " Jando", Part I, reprint from *Journal of the Royal Anthropological Institute*, 78, p. 159–68.

—1951b, "Jando", Part II, reprint from *Journal of the Royal Anthropological Institute*, p. 81–111.

—1957, "Gogo Law and Customs". Mimeograph.

Jacobson-Widding, A., 1979, *Red-White-Black as a Mode of Thought: A Study of Triadic Classification by Colours in the Ritual Symbolism and Cognitive Thought of the People of the Lower Congo*. Uppsala: Acta Universitatis Upsaliensis.

—1984, *Body Symbolism in Connection with the Relationship of Joking, Respect and Avoidance*. Uppsala: Department of Cultural Anthropology, University of Uppsala.

—1989, "Notion of Heat and Fever among the Manyika of Zimbabwe", in A. Jacobson-Widding and D. Westerlund (eds.), *Culture, Experience and Pluralism: Essays on African Ideas of Illness and Healing*. Uppsala: Acta Universitatis Uppsaliensis.

Lucas, S.A. and T.S. Tengo, 1975, *Utani na jamii Ukwere*. Nairobi: Foundation Books.

MacLean, S. and S. Efua Graham, 1983, *Female Circumcision, Excision and Infibulation: the Facts and Proposals for Change*. Report 47. London: Minority Rights Group.

Ntukula, M., 1994, "The Initiation Rite", in Z. Tumbo-Masabo and R. Liljeström (eds.), *Chelewa Chelewa. The Dilemma of Teenage Girls*. Uppsala: Scandinavian Institute of African Studies.

Slack, A.T., 1988, "Female Circumcision: a Critical Appraisal", *Human Rights Quarterly*, 10, 437–86.

"Tanzania: Circumcision still rampant", *Win News*, Winter 1993, 40–1.

Toubia, N., 1994, "Female Circumcision as a Public Health Issue", *The New England Journal of Medicine*, 331, 712–15.

Tumbo-Masabo, Z., 1994, "Too little too late", in Z. Tumbo-Masabo and R. Liljeström (eds.), *Chelewa, Chelewa. The Dilemma of Teenage Girls*. Uppsala: Scandinavian Institute of African Studies.

Walker, A., 1993, *Warrior Marks: Female Genital Mutilation and the Sexual Blinding of Women*. New York: Harcourt Brace.

Chapter 5
Teenage Mothers in their Second Pregnancies

Rosalia S. Katapa

Teenage motherhood is a problem in almost all developing countries. "The problems and characteristics associated with adolescent fertility, such as health, early marriage, low labour force participation and high child morality, are not so different from one poor country to another" (Kandiah, 1989). Demographic and health surveys show that there is widespread teenage motherhood in sub-Saharan countries. They also show that a proportion of teenagers, some of them unmarried, have had two or three births and that others are in their second and third pregnancies.

Table 1 below is extracted from the *Tanzania Demographic and Health Survey (TDHS) report*. The TDHS was conducted between October 1991 and March 1992.

Table 1. *Numbers of children born to teenagers in the TDHS sample*

Teenagers' 15–19 years	Number of children born				sample size
	0	1	2	3	
% of teenagers	76.8	19.7	3.4	0.1	2,183
% married teenagers	42.1	48.4	9.0	0.5	558

The previous studies by our team (Tumbo-Masabo and Liljeström, 1994) have shown how teenage girls are unprepared for motherhood when they fall pregnant. Tumbo-Masabo concludes that teenage girls get information on reproduction when it is too late and they are already pregnant. I have documented the socioeconomic and health problems which face teenage mothers in arranged marriages. Most of the problems were expressed by teenage wives themselves. Other chapters present problems which confront unmarried teenagers during their first pregnancies, their deliveries, and as young mothers. Given the documented problems, one would expect that a teenage mother would delay another pregnancy until she is mature enough and economically independent.

In places like the USA, abortion is one of the solutions to teenage pregnancies: "More than one million teenagers become pregnant each year in the United States, and about half of them give birth" (Freeman and Rickels, 1993). In many developing countries, including Tanzania, abortion is illegal so that teenage pregnancy almost always means teenage childbirth. A study in the USA observed that closeness to a boyfriend/father of first child was a contributing factor in second pregnancies (Freeman and Rickels, 1993).

In the current study I was concerned to identify the socio-economic and cultural conditions that contribute to teenage mothers' second pregnancies. I made four assumptions, namely:

- Teenage mothers find themselves pregnant because of the failure of family planning methods they use;
- Before the second pregnancy, teenagers marry men who are not the fathers of their firstborn;
- Teenagers whose first babies did not survive decide to become pregnant again; and
- Teenage mothers seek sex in order to get financial and/or material support from the men they go out with. In the process they fall pregnant.

The young mothers were asked questions on their educational level, source of income, religion, marital status, marital expectations, housing amenities, and the welfare of the first child. A teenager who qualified for being interviewed in this research had to have the following characteristics:

- she should not have attained 20 on the first contact day;
- she should be in her second pregnancy or have had two births; and
- she should have been unmarried when her first child was born.

My research areas were Manzese in Dar es Salaam city and Mwanjelwa in Mbeya municipality. The two areas have much in common. They both started as suburbs and slums. With the growth of Dar es Salaam and Mbeya, they are now large, densely populated urban slums. These areas are centres of poverty and criminal activity.

The teenagers were identified through ten-cell leaders. Ten cell-leaders are the lowest leaders in the country's administrative structure. A ten-cell leader is in charge of ten compounds/households in the community. The ten-cell leader was asked if there was any teenager in the cell who qualified for the study. Once a respondent had been identified, an appointment was made with her.

Two questionnaires were designed, one for interviewing married teenage mothers and the other the unmarried ones.

Who were they?

There were twenty-one respondents, fourteen of them in Manzese and the other seven in Mwanjelwa. Their ages ranged from 18 to almost 20 years. Ten of them were Christians; all the Mwanjelwa respondents were Christian. The remaining eleven were Muslims, one of them having converted from Christianity to Islam through marriage.

All of the twenty-one teenage mothers had been to school. Thirteen of them had completed primary school. Two others had gone to secondary schools although only one of them completed secondary school. The remaining six teenage mothers had dropped out of school for different reasons. This had happened between Standards 2 and 6.

When the teenage mothers became pregnant for the first time, the parents of eleven of them were still married while those of six others were either divorced or separated. Three others had each lost one parent. At that time, six of them were living with both parents and eleven others were living either with a mother or a sister.

The ages of the firstborn of the teenage mothers ranged from 2 to 6 years. Five teenage mothers were in their second pregnancies and the other sixteen had already had two births.

Four assumptions

Research findings indicate that the four assumptions are valid.

Assumption 1: Teenage mothers find themselves pregnant because of the failure of the family planning methods they use.

Two of the seven married teenage mothers in Manzese had been pregnant twice before marriage. Both of them claimed that both the pregnancies were due to failure of the family planning methods they were using. One of them was on the pill which she acquired from a pharmacy. The other one was using a traditional method of wearing a herb (*kuvaa dawa*), given to her by her grandmother.

Another two of the seven unmarried teenage mothers in Manzese were on the pill when they became pregnant for the second time. One of them had obtained the pill from a pharmacy and the other one from a maternal and child health (MCH) clinic. Two other teenage mothers in Mwanjelwa claimed that they were on the pill when they became pregnant again, and they had both acquired the pill from the Family Planning Association of Tanzania (UMATI).

It is concluded that six teenage mothers claimed that the family planning methods they had been using had let them down. They were among eleven teenage mothers who claimed to have used the pill after the birth of their firstborn.

Assumption 2: Before the second pregnancy, teenagers marry men who are not the fathers of their firstborn.

The research yielded eight married teenage mothers who were unmarried at the birth of their firstborn children.

Six teenage mothers had married men who were not the fathers of their firstborns. Of the six, two had been on the pill before marriage. They stopped using the pill upon marriage in the hope of falling pregnant. Two others were neither pregnant nor on the pill at the time of marriage. The four teenage mothers became pregnant within one year of marriage. The remaining two of the six teenage mothers got married when they were in their second pregnancies.

On the other hand, one teenager who married her firstborn's father had a second pregnancy almost three years after her marriage. This could be because she already had a child by him. It is possible that once a teenage mother marries a man who is not the father of her child, she feels duty bound to bear another child, perhaps to ensure the security of her marriage.

Assumption 3: Teenagers decide to become pregnant again because their first babies did not survive.

Two of the fourteen Manzese teenage mothers had lost their firstborns before falling pregnant again. One of them was already married at the time of this research. Her firstborn had died of measles at the age of five months. Seven months later the mother had a church wedding to a man who was not the father of her late child and one month later she became pregnant. At the time of this research, she was in her second pregnancy. The other was an unmarried teenager who had been expelled from school because she had fallen pregnant. She had been in Standard 6. Her father had been so angry that he had taken her to a police station. The man responsible for the pregnancy disappeared from sight. Late in the year, she gave birth to a baby boy. The child died of a fever one year and a half later. After the birth of her first child she went on the pill. When her child died, she stopped using the pill because she wanted to become pregnant. At the time of this research, she was still pregnant.

In Mwanjelwa, a married teenager and another unmarried one had lost their firstborns before becoming pregnant again. The married teenager had a customary marriage late in 1993. Early in the following year she had lost her one-year-old child, who had died of stomach problems (*ndonda*). She did not indulge in sex after the birth and before the death of her first child. At the time of this research, she was in her second pregnancy. The unmarried teenager lost her child six months after it was born: this was in 1989. The child had died of fever. By then the teenager had already lost her father and was living with her mother. Her second pregnancy was not planned.

This assumption cannot be rejected, particularly if we carefully evaluate the case of the Manzese unmarried teenager who stopped using the pill on the death of her first child so that she could become pregnant.

Assumption 4: Teenage mothers seek sex in order to get financial or material support from men, and in the process they fall pregnant.

One Mwanjelwa teenage mother indicated that money might have been the cause of her second pregnancy. She said, "*Ni wakati mwingine nasema labda nikatafute hela ya sabuni kumbe ndio napata mimba ya pili*" which means there are times when you say "Let me go and look for money to buy soap that you get a second pregnancy." During focus group discussions in Manzese, it was stated that economic hardship compelled some teenage girls and mothers to look for men who would provide them with financial and/or material support.

It is possible that some men use the poverty of teenage mothers as a means of luring them without the teenage mothers realizing that they are being trapped. The Mwanjelwa unmarried teenage mother we mentioned was a victim of this strategy. She had lost her father and was living with her poor mother. A certain man made her pregnant, but when he was called to confess before her relatives, he refused. Since then the man has started evading her. She had a child and six months later it died. One year after that the man resurfaced and made every possible excuse for his long absence. He also gave her money. She became pregnant again. When he was summoned by her relatives, he denied all responsibility for the pregnancy. At the end of the discussion with the teenager, she said, *"Tamaa ya pesa za yule bwana zikaniponza ikaingia mimba bila ya kuitaka"* meaning "My attraction to that man's money led me falsely into an unplanned pregnancy."

Similarly, another Mwanjelwa unmarried teenage mother became pregnant again because the first child's father resurfaced, showered her with presents, and demanded that she bear him another child. He promised that he would take care of her and the children financially. She became pregnant again and later had a second child. He kept his promise by providing her with some money.

Parents' reaction to daughters' pregnancies

Parents and guardians of all twenty-one teenage mothers were annoyed when they learned that their daughters were pregnant (first pregnancies). All of them demanded to know who the men were responsible for the pregnancies. The actions taken thereafter differed. In one case, the stepfather chased away his wife together with her daughter. He asserted that he was not ready to take care of someone else's daughter and someone else's child. In another case, as already noted, the daughter was taken to a police station. In several other cases, the men responsible for the pregnancies had been summoned to face the girls' parents, and some of them never responded. In other cases, the daughter was told to leave home and go to live with the man who was responsible for the pregnancy, only to come back and inform her parents that the man had refused to receive her.

Many parents and guardians felt dismayed and helpless when they realized that their daughters were pregnant once again. The following quotations signify this feeling. One young mother said, *"Baba alisema sikuulizi tena, hata la kufanya nashindwa na mtoto wewe"*, i.e.,"My father said he was not going to ask me anything because he was fed up with me." Another said her parents had told her *"Kazi kwako"* which means "That is your problem". A third one said *"Walinika-sirikia na kunirudisha kijijini"* meaning "They were angry and returned me to our home village".

To summarize, the daughters' second pregnancies came as a shock to many parents, who thought that their daughters had learned their lesson from their first pregnancies. In other words, most parents had expected their daughters would be "good girls" and not fall pregnant a second time.

Paternity of children

A breakdown of the paternity of the teenage mothers' children is made in Table 2.

Table 2. *Paternity of the two children*

	Do both children have the same father?		
	Yes	No	
Married mothers	2	6	
Unmarried mothers	7	6	
Total	9	12	21

Note: They were all unmarried when their first children were born.

It is clear that only two teenage mothers had married their firstborns' fathers, one of them being in a "forced marriage" (*ndoa ya mkeka*). The second one was married to the man because his parents and relatives convinced him to marry her.

Apart from these two teenagers, the rest of the married teenage mothers were not living with their firstborns. Instead, these children were living with their maternal grandparents. Some of the unmarried teenage mothers were living in their parents' homes with their children. A few others were living in rented single rooms, but their firstborns were with their maternal grandparents. Only two firstborns of unmarried teenage mothers were living with their fathers.

It is thus concluded that most of the time the burden of bringing up the children of teenage mothers is born by the teenagers' parents. Moreover, many fathers do not contribute to the upkeep of their out-of-wedlock children. In addition to the four fathers who were living with their children, only two others were assisting in the upkeep of their children. Their assistance was voluntary.

Teenage mothers' feelings towards their men

Most of the unmarried teenage mothers seemed to be on good terms with their men (fathers of the second born, if different from that of the firstborn), despite the fact that the men did not contribute much or anything to the upkeep of the children. To a certain extent, this appears to be risky for a third pregnancy might the outcome of this continuing friendship. Alternatively, it might be a road leading to marriage. Two teenagers, however, had different stories to tell. The father of the two children of a Mwanjelwa teenager was transferred to Dodoma, and that was the end of communication between the two parents. The father of the second born of a Manzese teenager ran away by changing residences within Dar es Salaam. She has never seen him since.

Economic status of teenage mothers

The unmarried teenage mothers' economic standing was not good. In Manzese, all the unmarried teenage mothers except two were unemployed and not engaged in any economic activity. As a result, they were leading lives of poverty. One teenage mother who was living with her widowed mother said, *"Wakati mwingine tulikuwa hatujui tutakula nini"* meaning "Sometimes we did not even know where our next meal would come from." This was in response to a question about her economic activities after the birth of her firstborn and before her second pregnancy. The two exceptions included the one who was employed. The second one was a *"mama ntilie"*, that is, engaged an informal economic activity of cooking and selling food in the open or on makeshift sites. The shared characteristic between the two teenage mothers is that they both had migrated from upcountry.

In Mwanjelwa, all the unmarried teenage mothers were involved in informal economic activities. They were not rich but they were able to keep busy and to obtain an income. They were involved in frying and selling buns and rice buns (*maandazi na vitumbua*), buying rice, beans, finger millet, and milk wholesale and selling it retail. Indeed, informal economic activities have no entry qualifications. As a result, among those who enter competition is very stiff. Fatu, who lived with her parents, told that sometimes she had to return home with her unsold buns and take them to the marketplace the following day. By then they would be stale. If they were not bought that day either, she would let her siblings eat them.

About half of married teenage mothers were economically active. One of them was employed. Three other Manzese teenage mothers were involved in informal economic activities. The activities were

making and selling "ice cream" as well as selling groundnuts, frying
and selling buns, and buying charcoal wholesale and selling it retail.
The Mbeya married teenage mother made and sold buns. Before her
marriage and her second pregnancy, she used to sell poor quality rice
(*chenga*) at the grinding and hauling mills.

Prospects of marriage

In the study, the teenage mothers indicated if they were married or
not. The different types of marriages are presented in Table 3.

Table 3. *Types of marriages among teenage mothers*

Type of marriage	Frequency
Muslim	3
Muslim (*ndoa ya mkeka*—"forced marriage")	1
Cohabiting	2
Customary	1
Christian	1
Total	8

All eight teenage mothers were in monogamous marriages. Three of
the six non-cohabiting teenage mothers had married divorced men.

Once again, the definition of marriage appears to be problematic.
Two Manzese cohabiting teenage mothers considered themselves to
be married, so they filled out questionnaires meant for married
teenagers. On the other hand, one Mwanjelwa and two other Manzese
teenage mother who were cohabiting did not consider themselves to
be married, and filled questionnaires meant for unmarried girls. One
cohabiting teenage mother who considered herself as being married
informed us that she had forced the cohabitation. Her words were,
*"Nilifosi. Nilihamia kidogo kidogo bila ya yeye mwenyewe kujua. Alishitukia
tayari nimejijenga"*, which means "I forced the cohabition by moving in
slowly, cautiously, and not letting him know my motive."

In many patrilineal societies in Tanzania, teenage mothers do not
have as much choice of future husbands as teenage girls without children. Moreover, most societies are Christian, and hold true the view
that there should be one-man one-wife "till God does us part". Many
young men feel more comfortable in marrying teenage girls rather
than teenage mothers. The responses on whether teenage mothers, in

general, had the same chances of marriage as teenage girls are presented in Table 4.

Table 4. *Marriage market*

Do teenage mothers have the same chances of marriage as teenage girls?

Respondents		Response	
		Yes	No
Married teenage mothers		4	4
Unmarried teenage mothers in:			
	Manzese	2	4
	Mwanjelwa	0	6
Total		6	14

Three of the four married teenage mothers and the two unmarried ones who replied yes said it all depended on one's luck and were from Manzese. The fourth married teenage mother who replied yes was from Mwanjelwa, and she said this could happen in villages if a teenage mother was of good behaviour. The four married teenage mothers who replied no said that most men do not like to take care of other men's children.

It can be seen that a majority of unmarried teenage mothers believe that teenage mothers have lower chances of marriage than girls. This to a certain extent is a sign of despair (*kukata tamaa*) among the teenage mothers. This can lead to their continuing to bear children out-of wedlock. The reasons given by the majority of the unmarried teenage mothers for having lower chances of marriage were that:

- Men do not like to take care of other men's children;
- Even if a man marries a teenage mother who leaves her child with her parents, the man will still dislike his wife's visits to her parents;
- The economy is very bad and many people are financially distressed. In addition to not wanting to see the other man's children in his compound, a man does not like to commit his finances to them, e.g., in terms of clothes, school fees, food, and medication;
- A teenage mother appears older and shabbier than a girl, i.e., a girl appears more attractive than a teenage mother; and
- If a man marries a teenage mother, his friends will laugh at him for marrying an old "used" woman (*ameoa mtumba*).

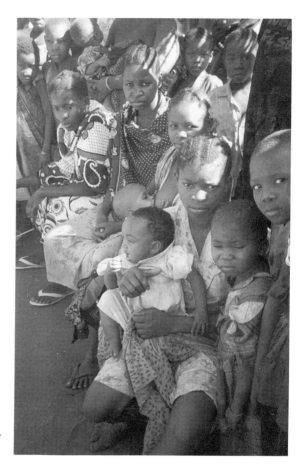

Previously it was alright to marry a woman with out-of-wedlock children. Due to the current economic hardship, nobody wants to take care of someone else's children.

(Photo Rita Liljeström)

A teenage mother from a matrilineal society said that previously it was allright in their society to marry a woman with out-of-wedlock children. However, due to the current economic hardship, nobody now wants to take care of someone else's children.

Finally, despite the fact that most teenage mothers with two children or in their second pregnancies despaired of marriage, they still had social support from their kin. For example, most of their firstborns were living with and depending on the mother's parents. Some of the teenage mothers were also dependent on their parents, which included living with them and getting most of their financial and material support from them.

Focus group discussions

Focus group discussions were held in Manzese and Mwanjelwa. Teenage mothers of two or who were in their second pregnancies participated.

The conditions identified as contributing to teenage second pregnancies are:

- Economic: some teenage mothers are left on their own with their children (firstborns). Being unemployed and having no source of income, they are compelled to look for men so that they can receive financial and/or material support.
- False promises from men were also causes of second pregnancies. This has two facets. One is the resurfacing of the teenager's boyfriend (father of the first child) who reassures her that he is back in her life, and will never leave her again. After making her pregnant, he runs away again. The other having a new boyfriend who assures her that he is not as bad as her former boyfriend (father of the first child) who had run away after making her pregnant. He also makes her pregnant and runs away!;
- Some teenage mothers are "sexually weak". They do not want a day or several days to pass without their having sexual intercourse; and
- Some teenagers are encouraged by their parents' attitudes. There are parents who do not care whether their daughters go out with men.

The feelings and reactions of parents, relatives and neighbours upon realizing that a teenage mother is pregnant for a second time are:

- In some societies, becoming pregnant again while still at home creates a very bad impression. Some relatives and people in the neighbourhood privately tease the teenager's father by saying "Maybe be he is the one who makes her pregnant! How can he continue to have her in the home?" This is just sarcasm; they know he is innocent. The sarcastic words put pressure on the teenager's father who eventually expels her from his home;
- In some societies, it is a blessing, because children belong to the mother. In some other societies, people feel it is misbehaviour on the part of the teenage mother;

- Some people feel that if the man responsible for the second child is the father of the first child, then the man and woman are in love. Otherwise the teenage mother is regarded as a prostitute; and
- Some people believe that she has despaired of marriage, and that she has decided to reproduce so as to attain the size of family she believes to be desirable.

The Manzese and Mwanjelwa teenage mothers had the same experiences and feelings about the ineffectiveness of the legal system when it comes to the father's contribution to child maintenance. The Manzese group said the legal system fails them. The process is lengthy and cumbersome, and discourages them. This view was summarized thus: When you go to court you are told "come tomorrow" and when you go again you are told "come the day after tomorrow". Many adjournments take place and at times you are told "bring witnesses". The Mwanjelwa group said that the most discouraging aspect is that once a teenage mother takes her man to court, she is told to come again on such and such date. This process of "come again on such and such a date" continues. If the teenage mother persistently goes to court on the set dates, more often than not court elders or other elders take her aside and seriously warn her that her child could die as a result of her persistence. Once a teenage mother gets such a warning, she may believe that some bad people may decide that the child is the cause of the court "battle", and that if the child "exits" the world, the "battle" will be over. They may then bewitch the child so that it dies.

The two groups also shared feelings on the arrogance of former boyfriends (fathers of their children). According to the Manzese group, teenage mothers sometimes become discouraged from taking legal action by what the other partners say: For example, a male partner could say "I was not the only one going out with her when she became pregnant. How can I know that the child is mine?" Similarly, the Mwanjelwa group said some men make very rude comments when they are called by ten-cell leaders to effect a reconciliation. Such comments commonly include "I was not the only boyfriend, she had many of us", or "How do I knew the child is mine when many of us were sharing her?" They also say that "sometimes, at the meeting convened by the ten-cell leader, the man agrees that he will provide support". To start with, he may give the teenage mother 2,000 shillings (equivalent to four US dollars). When approached again, he says "I have no money" or "I am unemployed, so where do you expect me to get money from?"

Stories of failure and success

I will share some mothers' stories of failure and success.

Nasemba

Nasemba was born in 1974 in a Christian home in Kilimanjaro region. Five months before finishing her secondary school education in Dar es Salaam, she realized she was pregnant. That was in 1992. Fearing that the pregnancy would be detected, she asked for permission from the school authorities to be a day scholar rather than a boarder student. Upon obtaining this permission, she moved to the home of her brother, who was her guardian.

As a day student, Nasemba tried hard to hide her pregnancy so that she would not be detected and expelled from school. She succeeded in her mission and she told us that *"Japokuwa nilikuwa na mimba, nilijitahidi kuificha ili nimalize shule, Mungu alinisaidia"* meaning "I succeeded in hiding my pregnancy and God helped me".

When Nasemba's parents in Kilimanjaro region heard of her pregnancy, they were angry. By then, she had already finished school. The man who made her pregnant was from her tribe. During their friendship, there had been promises of marriage. Hopes of marriage vanished when she became pregnant. She gave birth to a healthy baby boy who died of measles five months later.

After the child's death, Nasemba gained employment and later a steady boyfriend. They married in church early in February 1994. Asked about contraceptives, Nasemba said she had never used them. Nasemba and her husband were living in a reasonably good house which had water and electricity.

Nasemba's story is one of misfortune and success. Falling pregnant in school was a misfortune, hiding it till she finished school five months later a success. Losing her baby five months later was a misfortune. Getting a job, a husband, and falling pregnant again, which she had been longing for, can be considered as successes.

Akani

Akani was born in 1974 in Zambia. Her parents were Tanzanians but from different tribes. Her father died when she was very young. She dropped out of school when she was in Standard 2 the reason being that her mother could not afford to buy school uniforms.

When Akani fell pregnant for the first time she was living with her sister in Mwanjelwa. Her sister became so annoyed that she hardly talked to Akani. Akani gave birth to a healthy baby girl. After the birth of the child, Akani started engaging in an income generating activity in order to buy necessities for herself and her child. She sold low quality rice which is later ground into flour for making rice buns. The man who had made her pregnant never assisted her financially or materially. The child died of stomach problems (*ndonda*) at the age of one year.

After the child's death, Akani became a devoted Assemblies of God Christian. She and her mother had been Moravians. It was while she was at her new church that she met her husband, a divorcee. The man paid about 5,000 shillings (about 10 US dollars) as an advance on bridewealth. They then started living together as husband and wife. Living together can be considered as customary marriage, because part of the bridewealth has been paid and her "parents" had consented.

Upon marriage, Akani changed her occupation from that of selling poor quality rice to that of making and selling buns. After the birth and before the death of her first child, Akani did not indulge in sex, so the question of contraceptive use was irrelevant. When she started living with her husband, she did not use contraceptives because she wanted to fall pregnant. When we last visited Akani, she was seven months pregnant. She and her husband were living in a house without electricity or water. She was using firewood for cooking and kerosene for lighting their open lamp (*kibatari*).

Mwanakombo

Mwanakombo was born in 1975 in Dar es Salaam. She finished her primary school education in 1989. Mwanakombo's parents were Muslims. They had divorced while she was still young. After the divorce, each parent had continued to live in Dar es Salaam. Mwanakombo was brought up by her mother.

Early in 1990, Mwanakombo became pregnant. She gave birth to a healthy girl towards the end of the year. She continued to live with her mother during the pregnancy and after delivery. Talking of her life after the first birth, she said it had been hard because her mother was neither married nor employed.

Mwanakombo never stopped seeing her man after the first birth. She used oral contraceptives, the pill, to prevent another pregnancy. One day in 1993, Mwanakombo and her boyfriend were surprised while having sexual intercourse (*walifumaniwa*). Her father called a sheikh who married Mwanakombo and her boyfriend there and then, her father paying the sheikh's fees. In Kiswahili this type of marriage is called "*ndoa ya mkeka*", it is in a sense a forced marriage, for neither the bride nor the groom are prepared for it. No bridewealth was paid for Mwanakombo because the marriage was a sudden one. Under normal circumstances of "*ndoa ya mkeka*", bridewealth is given later. I wonder if this will be the case for Mwanakombo because her husband is poor. He is a young man in his early twenties.

Mwanakombo stopped taking the pill after her marriage. She became pregnant and had her second child in December 1993. Mwanakombo is on very good terms with both her parents and her in-laws.

Mwanakombo and her husband are living a poverty; they do not have any economic activity to sustain them. Mwanakombo's mother has been selling charcoal for years. She would buy a sack of charcoal, open it and divide the charcoal into small amounts. She would then sell each amount separately (retail). She would retain the capital and use the profit for buying foodstuffs and bare essentials. Before her marriage, Mwanakombo used to assist her mother in this business. After her marriage, she and her husband help her with the business. It is from this business that they survive. Sometimes the money they earn in a day is not enough to buy food for two households, and as a result Mwanakombo, her husband, and their two children end up eating at her mother's home. They live in a small hut (*banda*) which does not have electricity or water. Despite the poverty, Mwanakombo and her husband are still in love and respect each other.

Kedekede

Kedekede was born in 1974 in Ifakara, Morogoro region. She was born of Muslim parents. In 1988, she finished her primary education in Ifakara. She then moved to Dar es Salaam to live with her sister.

While in Dar es Salaam, Kedekede fell in love with a young man from Lindi, i.e. a Mwera. Kedekede became pregnant, and her boyfriend asked to marry her. Kedekede's parents, who were still in Ifakara, refused the marriage proposal because he came from Lindi which was too far away from them. Kedekede gave birth to a baby boy in 1990. Their love kept flourishing despite the marriage refusal by Kedekede's parents.

About one year after the birth of her child, Kedekede obtained employment. After some time, she rented a room and started to live on her own, i.e., she became independent. Kedekede kept on seeing her boyfriend from Lindi and by mid-1993, she had conceived again. Kedekede's boyfriend once again approached her parents with a marriage proposal and they refused for the same reasons as before.

When we visited Kedekede, her second child was six months old. The 4-year-old firstborn was living with Kedekede's elder sister. We were told that her boyfriend from Lindi was very close to her and still wanted to marry her, despite her parents repeated refusals. Our observation was that the boyfriend had almost moved in with her. It appears that Kedekede's parents we re fighting a losing battle.

Kedekede's economic status was not bad, because she was employed. She had rented a room in a house with no electricity or water. She was dressed well and her baby looked healthy. Her boyfriend was also employed.

Binzari

Binzari was born in 1975 in Dar es Salaam. Her parents are both Christian. Binzari belongs to a matrilineal tribe which is centred in southern Tanzania. Binzari's father was a watchman at a construction site. The whole family was living at the site.

Binzari dropped out of school in 1990 when she was in Standard 6. The reason for this was pregnancy. She had been made pregnant by one of the teenage boys in the neighbourhood. When her father realized that Binzari was pregnant he followed the boy and threatened him by telling him that he would have to marry her or be taken to court, because Binzari was still a schoolgirl. The teenage boy compromised by promising that he would take care of her financially and materially.

Binzari gave birth to a baby boy in the same year that she had dropped out of school. At the birth of her first child, Binzari was anaemic and the baby had a very low birth weight (*njiti*). She and the baby stayed at Muhimbili hospital for two months.

Binzari continued to see her boyfriend after the birth of her baby. She was using oral contraceptives, i.e., the pill, which she obtained from a maternal and child health (MCH) clinic. Early in 1993, Binzari discovered that she was pregnant again. *"Vidonge vilinikataa"* was her reply when asked whether she had planned the pregnancy. The reply means that Binzari fell pregnant while she was still on the pill. She gave birth to her second child in September 1993.

At the time we visited Binzari in mid-1994, she and her two children were still living with and depending on her parents. She claimed that her boyfriend was contributing very little to the upkeep of their children, despite the fact that she was providing him with all conjugal services. *"Hataki kunioa ingawa huduma za unyumba nampa, anasema atalea watoto"*, was Binzari's reply when asked whether they were expecting to get married. The reply means that he has categorically refused to marry her although he continues to have sexual intercourse with her.

Discussion

I have presented some socioeconomic and cultural aspects affecting teenage mothers of two children or who are in their second pregnancies. We have seen that there are many conditions which lead to second pregnancies among teenagers. Among them are failure or improper use of contraceptive pills, marriage to a man who is not the father of the teenager's first child, non-survival of the first child, and looking for financial and material support from men.

From Table 2 above, we conclude that men do not generally marry teenagers by whom they have already had children. Culture plays a significant role in determining whether a man marries the mother of his child or not. We have three examples to demonstrate this conclusion. The first is when the young man is forced into a marriage (*ndoa ya mkeka*) by the teenage mother's father. As a Muslim, the young man respected this marriage just as every other man might his own voluntary marriage. A second pregnancy occured and a child was born to the "forced" marriage. The teenage wife (Mwanakombo) and her husband respect each other as other husbands and wives do. *Ndoa ya mkeka* is not a rare form of marriage. Parents get tired of seeing young men spoiling their daughters. So they spy on the movements of their daughters. As soon as they catch the couple indulging in sexual intercourse, there is no choice but marriage. Parents of the teenage girl/mother call a sheikh who conducts the marriage. The parents pay the sheikh's fee. After that the couple is expected to live like any other couple and the husband is expected to provide bridewealth.

The second example involving culture is that of a man from Mara region who was convinced by his relatives to marry the mother of his child. Indeed, this man comes from a place where they respect their "blood" and hence are not prepared to lose it by neglecting out-of-wedlock children. Thus the man married the young mother of the child of his blood.

A new kind of cultural conflict arises when marriage is no longer a bond between clans but a contract between two persons, as in the case of Kedekede. Thus reminds us of what is involved in and expected of marriage. Kedekede was torn between her culture, which is highly respected and closely followed by her parents, and her lover from another tribe. We cannot blame Kedekede for being in love with a man from faraway Lindi; people say "love is blind". Neither can we blame Kedekede's parents and clan for refusing the marriage proposal; they were respecting and observing their culture. Practically, in most African societies, marriage is not just a contract between two people, but is between two clans. The advantages of a daughter marrying nearby are:

- The two clans know each other when problems arise;
- The two clans assist each other when problems arise;
- The two clans join hands in celebrations. For example, suppose Kedekede was to marry into her tribe. After some time when Kedekeke's brother marries, her husbands' clan would contribute to Kedekede's clan to make the wedding festival a success;
- In general the "family" is extended because the bride's and groom's clans "merge";
- The couple gets moral and material support from clans on both sides; and
- If the daughter dies and leaves children, her clan will continue to provide moral and material support to them. Consequently, the children will have both parents' clans to socialize with and be supported by.

Indeed, once a daughter marries far away, all the above advantages are lost. Many parent are particularly concerned about how to assist their daughter in cases of problems or illness if she marries and lives far away. Also of great concern is the "loss of grandchildren" if she dies where she is married. We conclude that it is out of love for their daughter that Kedekede's parents refuse the marriage proposal of the man from distant Lindi. This was a dilemma for Kedekede who was residing in cosmopolitan Dar es Salaam, where cultural attachments are weak and her boyfriend from Lindi was just nearby.

It appears that economic hardships are scaring young men away from marriage. At the same time, economic hardships are making teenage girls and mothers vulnerable to men. The consequences are quite clear: pregnancies out-of-wedlock, and sexually transmitted diseases, including AIDS.

Idleness among both young men and teenage girls is the biggest factor which contributes to teenage pregnancies. Most teenage mothers were made pregnant by young men. Most of these girls were more or less idle, as were the young men. Unemployment is quite high and it has hit young men hardest. About 80 per cent of the youths who complete primary education (seven years in school) are left with nothing to do. Despite being energetic, they are left idle! It is common to see groups of youths sitting in "jobless corners" with nothing to do except crack jokes and comment on the physical features of girls who pass by. We conclude that as long as the economic situation of the country continues to be gloomy, more and more youths will be left idle and the outcome will be an increase in unplanned teenage motherhood. The real victims of this dilemma are the parents of teenage mothers, they are the ones who must take care of their teenage daughters' children.

In focus group discussions, from answers to the question "What factors contribute to teenage mothers indulging in sexual intercourse?", it appears that teenage mothers cannot differentiate between indulging in sexual intercourse and becoming pregnant. This compels us to believe that birth control education has not reached many teenagers. Birth control would allow a teenage mother to indulge in sexual intercourse without becoming pregnant, and a second pregnancy would be prevented.

It is common knowledge that some teenagers, girls and mothers, consent with "sugar daddies". Our research did not manage to identify any teenage mother whose man-friend was a "sugar daddy".

What could be the reasons? It has been stated that Manzese and Mwanjelwa are poor and crimeridden areas. Maybe "sugar daddies" do not want their teenage girlfriends come from such areas.

The burden of providing for grandchildren born-out-of wedlock continues to be heavy for the parents of the teenage mother. Formal courts were not seen as an effective means of obliging the men to share responsibility for their children. The cycle of ignorance, the cultural crisis, and poverty continue to trap young girls into successive pregnancies in early womanhood, while the fathers tend to run away.

References

Freeman, E.W. and K. Rickels, 1993, *Early Child Bearing: Perspectives of Black Adolescents on Pregnancy, Abortions and Contraceptions*. Newbury Park: Saga Publications.

Kandiah, V., 1989, "Child Bearing by Women under Twenty Worldwide". Notes from the seminar series: The Determinants and Consequences of Female Headed Households. The Population Council and International Center for Research on Women.

Katapa, R.S., 1994, "Arranged marriages", in Z. Tumbo-Masabo and R. Liljeström (eds.), *Chelewa, Chelewa. The Dilemma of Teenage Girls*. Uppsala: Scandinavian Institute of African Studies.

Tanzania Demographic and Health Survey 1991/92. A report. Dar es Salaam and Columbia: Bureau of Statistics, 1993.

Tumbo-Masabo, Z., 1994, "To little too late", in Z. Tumbo-Masabo and R. Liljeström (eds.), *Chelewa, Chelewa. The Dilemma of Teenage Girls*. Uppsala: Scandinavian Institute of African Studies.

ANNEX TO CHAPTER 5

RECOMMENDATIONS

Training

Folk Development Centres should be increased so as to equip youths with skills to engage in self-employment. This will keep them busy and they will also improve their economic status. Many of them will not find time to engage in sex and will avoid unplanned parenthood.

Family planning education

Family planning education should be provided to youths. In particular after delivery of the first child, a teenage mother should be thoroughly taught about how to prevent another early pregnancy.

Self-esteem

The self-esteem of teenage mothers should be fostered. They should not feel that they are the society's "rejects" or *mitumba*. This recommendation arises from a perception among teenage mothers that they had fewer chances of marriage than other teenage girls. They said a teenage mother looked old, untidy, dirty, shabby and was a *mitumba* (secondhand material). The society should be sensitized to acknowledge the problems of unmarried teenage mothers; in this way, people will have more positive attitudes towards them.

Nondependency on men

Teenage mothers should be discouraged from depending on men. This practice does not solve their economic problems; instead it aggravates them by leading to new pregnancies. One teenage mother said, "at times you go out looking for money to buy soap for washing the baby's diapers and in the process you become pregnant." It is clear that this development produces more problems than solutions. Instead of having one mouth to feed and one set of diapers to wash, you end up with two.

Chapter 6
Boys' Views on Sexuality, Girls, and Pregnancies

Juliana C. Mziray

Generally, boys in Tanzania, irrespective of their ethnic origin, tend to differ from girls in their views on sexual matters. Boys are freer to explore sex than girls. They are not so easily dismissed as promiscuous by the community. Obviously, they do not fall pregnant, hence their sexual behaviour is not publicly apparent. Correspondingly, many researchers concentrate on girls' sexual behaviour and related problems, forgetting the indispensable role boys play in impregnating girls. This led me to examine boys' perceptions of sexuality and their views on girls and teenage pregnancies.

The impetus to conduct this study also arose out my having lived in two communities with different customary outlooks on teenage sexuality. One of these was Keni Aleni area in Rombo district, Kilimanjaro region, the homeland of the Chagga tribe. The Chagga are a restrictive patrilineal society. Boys and girls were traditionally not allowed to engage in sex before marriage. The other community was in Gairo area in Morogoro region, where the Kaguru live. The Kaguru are a matrilineal and permissive tribe who allow boys and girls to start sexual activities while they are still very young. The two areas have undergone rapid societal changes. Both areas are growing as business centres, so that people's lifestyles are changing and their established moral order is being disturbed.

Keni Aleni is on the border between Tanzania and Kenya. Its traditional values are influenced by the intensified mixing of people from these two countries. Gairo is a small town between Morogoro and Dodoma municipalities. Big trucks move to and from the two towns, bringing a mix of people of various backgrounds. This has led to changes in how the Kaguru understand their world. The main occupation of residents in the two areas is farming.

Several studies have shown that teenage boys engage in sexual activities while still very young (Kamuzora, 1987). It sometimes hap-

pens that relationships between boys and girls result in teenage pregnancies. Girls who fall pregnant are expelled from school, according
to Tanzanian school regulations. This forced me to explore how boys
view the teenage girls' pregnancies; are they, for example, ready to
accept the single mothers in marriage? These are some of the questions that this study attempts to highlight.

I was concerned about teenage sexuality and particularly interested in comparing the boys' views on sexual matters in the two
communities. With those aims in mind I interviewed ten boys in each
village, Gairo and Keni Aleni. I picked those boys by simply walking
around the streets and talking to people: I found a group of boys
sitting in a tree shed at the roadside. I met them while eating at the
same table; I took part in a youth' discussion in the church; I approached boys who sold sugarcane or fruits or sundries; I met them in
the neighbourhood. I had chats with them and we agreed upon a time
for interviews. Some of the boys later called a friend to be interviewed. They were all 15 to 19 years old. I am a mother in my 50s and they
trusted me.

Gairo boys

Gairo is a medium-sized village. Prior to the construction of the
Morogoro–Dodoma highway in the 1980s, it was just a small settlement. The lack of any large town between Morogoro and Dodoma
forced lorry drivers to adopt Gairo as their resting place, because of its
central location. Heavy trucks and tankers are a common sight even
today. This concentration of passengers, mostly drivers and their
helpers, has led to the construction of modern guesthouses and
restaurants, an activity that continues.

Gairo village is still backward. In spite of a population of about
10,000 people, there are only two primary schools, one being a missionary school and the other a government school. The schools were
built in 1965 and 1980 respectively. There is no secondary school,
technical school, or any vocational training centre. The majority of
those with some education are primary school graduates.

Gairo has a public health centre with three medical assistants. It is
from here that all primary medical services, including Mother Health
clinics and family planning are offered. As in most health centres in
the country, primary health education is conducted every morning for
the patients before the receive treatment. Patients who require a doc-

tor's attention are transferred to Morogoro regional hospital (260 kilometres away) or Berega mission hospital (about 50 kilometres away).

Moreover, there is a post office without telephone services. The
National Bank of Commerce has a branch in Gairo with only a few
customers. There is no electricity in the area.

The weather in Gairo is normally windy and dry. There is a short
rainy season, leaving the area very arid. Common crops are sweet
potatoes, maize, and millet. Because of the climate, horticulture is not
practised, depriving Gairo peasants of an extra income. The low rain-
fall has led to sparse water sources for domestic use and livestock.
The village's water supply is very unreliable. There are pipelines
coming into the village, but these are in most cases dry because of the
drying out of the source. The drought was so serious in 1991 and 1992
that the government had to offer food relief to most families to save
them from starvation.

The youths' jobs include fetching water from a mission village
nearby and selling it in Gairo. The youths also collect firewood, and
building materials such as poles and thatching grass, from nearby
forests and sell them to local people. Businesses like shopkeeping,
restaurants, or guesthouses, etc., are run by people who come from
elsewhere and are not local inhabitants. Similarly, most of the em-
ployees in government offices, school teachers, police, bank clerks,
etc., are from outside as a consequence of the Gairo youths' lack of
education.

Most of the boys I interviewed in Gairo were from low-income
families. Their parents had little education. The family's low socio-
economic status affected the boys' schooling. I came across Sayi at a
market place where he was chatting to a shopkeeper. He described the
situation most of the boys in the village experience. He is 18 years and
jobless. His father had two wives. Sayi attended school near his home
because primary education is compulsory. He managed to reach Standard 5 only. He could not afford soap to wash his uniform and as a
result he was often punished. This made him a truant at school. He
sometimes absconded from school to do paid work in order to buy
soap for washing his clothes. He could not complete primary education. In his family, there are five boys. Only one of them managed to
finish primary education.

Many boys in Gairo are jobless and spend most of their time in
jobless corners called *Kijiweni*. The word *jiwe* means a stone, a dry
mass, nonconsumable, with no life in it, normally dormant. *Kijiweni* is

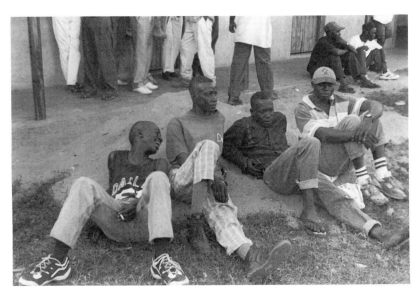

Kijiweni, the jobless corner   (Photo Benny Kisanga)

an informal meeting place, usually an open space used by the youths to spend their free time, free either because they are unemployed or have finished their daily activities.

Our youths, who are poorly educated and have no regular income meet at a suitable place on a street corner or under a tree to socialize among themselves. As they cannot afford to equip their meeting place with chairs and tables, they collect pieces of stone to sit on. They spend long hours there. People use to regard them as places to waste time or to discuss plans of unattainable action. I came to learn later that these jobless corners are not places where people spend time without any purpose, as the name suggests. A jobless corner is a place where boys exchange information on possible places to get work. They also discuss sexual matters. The corner is also some kind of bank where money is lent and where the boys can invite each other for an evening drink and other entertainment. Hence, *Kijiweni* means a lot to the Gairo boys.

Malenta from Gairo tells his story

Malenta is 18 years old and the firstborn of his mother, but fifthborn of his father, who has two wives. He enrolled in the nearby primary school in 1983 but left the school in Class 5. He was often beaten because of his dirty uniform or for missing school for several days without reason. His parents are farmers with low earnings. In most cases, there was no money for soap to wash his school uniform. Sometimes, Malenta missed school because he was generating income in order to help his mother buy food. Even now he has no reliable income. He works as a labourer for the trucks which carry heavy loads to town. Sometimes, he hires a bicycle and fetches water to sell or he works as labourer on other people's farms.

> I spend most of my time at *Kijiweni* where I meet most of my friends. We go there to refresh our minds after heavy work or when we are in severe financial straits (*mambo makali*). That is the only place where I can get someone to lend me money or give me a cigarette or get an invitation for an evening drink.

He commented on the changes associated with his maturity growing within the family.

> I can remember—under 7 years of age I knew the difference between boys and girls by the way they dress, their names and games. Girls usually play games like carrying stones on their backs and calling them children or they cook with pieces of clay pots. I liked girls more than boys. They are more gentle to deal with. As I grew older, let's say around 8 years, I used to see families holding large festivals for adolescent girls to announce that she had matured (*mwali*). At about 10 years girls in our class started looking like grown-up women. Their breasts become larger and their buttocks rounder. One day, I asked a senior boy the meaning of becoming *mwali*. He simply told me that when the girl has matured, she can give birth.

> Around Class 5, girls in our class, one after another, became *mwali*. By then we started to learn the science of the reproductive system, especially in animals. I came to understand that when external changes occur in female bodies, simultaneous changes also take place internally and that menarche is a confirmation of maturity.

> Several girls never completed primary education because of pregnancy. Few of them were lucky enough to deliver their children normally. Some had their children by means of an operation. Several girls lost their children and some of the children were very weak. I know two girls who lost their lives. One had tried to end pregnancy, and another died in pregnancy from a anaemia.

> My friendship with girls went through several stages. After graduating from initiation we formed a peer-group of seven boys. We decided to have girlfriends because at the initiation camp we were taught that a self-

respecting man must have a woman. We chose girls in our neighbour-hood and each of us matched ourself up with a girl. The matching was done by telling the young girls that we wanted to marry them. Usually the girl would react by beating you or crying. The main activity was joking or walking home from school together. We used to protect them from harassment by other boys. I would fight any boy who spoke nasty words to my girl.

At around 13 I started to have stronger feelings of love for girls. This time, I chose a girl near my house and tried to get close to her by talking in a friendly manner, but she never got the message and never reacted positively. In our peer-group, most talk by then was about girls. We talked about the way they dress, talk, or smile. Anything that a girl did was interesting to us; we would discuss it. A boy would claim that a certain girl had accepted him. Most often these were only lies. One would tell how he had danced with a girl at a local dance, another would relate how a girl had betrayed a certain boy and would gossip about who was in love with whom in the group.

To be accepted in a peer-group, you must talk about your activity with girls or else the other boys will look down on you, you will be considered weak or not presentable enough to attract a woman. There was also some speculation among members that if one does not have any sexual activity with a girl, then the man is sexually weak and is likely to become impotent. Wet dreams were considered a sign of a future bad disease. This is what made most of us start to involve ourselves in sexual play at an early age.

This time, I chose a girl on the basis of her appearance and shape. She was light skinned, tall, and slim. Her behaviour was not at all important at that time. I wrote a letter and gave it to my friend who handed it to her. I told her how much I was in love with her and could hardly sleep at night. I told her that she was the most beautiful girl in our area and I ended by telling her that I would love her forever. With such cunning words did she accept me. By then, I had already matured and I was very much troubled by the sexual feelings which caused me to indulge in strong relationships with girls. Most of my friends complained of such feelings—by 14 years, I assure you, no boy in this area is ignorant of sex play. I moved from one girl to another, causing conflicts among my friends and causing girls to fight. Once, I fell into the trap of venereal disease. I told one of my friends about my burning sensation and he laughed and said it was common in active men. He advised me to see a doctor who gave me some antibiotic pills and in a few days I was well again. I went on with this behaviour regardless of what happened. Once you start involving yourself in this game, you cannot avoid it. At about 16, I was a grown up. I started choosing girls according to their behaviour and dealt with them in a more mature manner. I went to discos and local dances with them. I would escort them home after a gathering, buy them presents, and visit their sick relatives. Nevertheless, I have not decided when to marry.

About unmarried girls in this area, I can say that they differ from one girl to another. I do not like the behaviour of most unmarried girls in our community. In recent years, strange and shocking behaviour has emerged. Unmarried girls move from their parent's residence and rent rooms somewhere, claiming that they want to live on their own. They are not employed and have no regular income-generating activities. They depend on men to meet their living expenses. As a result, they become prostitutes. Others stay in guesthouses with the truck drivers, who give them money to buy expensive dresses and heavy cosmetics. One result of this luxurious life is that other girls are attracted to it and start to behave the same way.

Most girls and even boys do not like hard work (farming). They want to live a leisurely life. This has rapidly increased the shameful acts in this area. Thefts and girls loitering on street corners at night and out-of-wedlock pregnancies are increasing. The community appears to accept them. There are other kinds of girls who move to town to look for employment. While in town, they do all sorts of bad things. Most of them will go home with out-of-wedlock babies or very sick and most are infected by HIV. Other girls brew and sell local beer until late at night. There have been cases where teenage girls have been beaten and badly injured by unknown men. Even, some married teenage girls divorce their husbands in order to live such a life. Lately, divorce cases in this area have become very high.

To me, if a girl has a steady boyfriend and falls pregnant, I feel comfortable provided the boy accepts his responsibility. If it is a girl who sells local beer or who goes to town with truck drivers, I am sure no one will accept her. I feel no sympathy for her. However, if after delivery she stays with her parents and takes care of the child, I would view her pregnancy as an accident although I myself would not marry such a woman. Several men are happily married to such women. I know girls of good behaviour. They stay with their parents, help them on the farm, and undertake some income-generating activities to meet their living expenses. They are satisfied with their income and have steady partners. Such girls will usually get married and raise happy families. This is the type of girls I can choose in marriage.

We have reached the point where Malenta finds himself in the present, but he adds a further comment.

There is a practice that I do not agree with. Teenage girls are allowed to use contraceptives. What for? Unmarried girls are not supposed to indulge in love play outside marriage. Allowing them to use pills means encouraging premarital sex.

Keni Aleni boys

Keni Aleni in Rombo district is a settlement on the southern slope of Mount Kilimanjaro, near the border of Kenya. Due because the roads are passable throughout the year, communication with nearby towns is very good, making business easy to conduct. Cross-border business between Tanzania and Kenya is increasing so much that Rombo has grown to be very well known for commerce and traffic.

Keni Aleni area has a population about 50,000 people. There are primary and secondary schools, a technical school, and a homecraft centre. There is a government-run health centre. Patients who require a doctor's attention are transferred to Mkuu government hospital or to Huruma hospital, which is run by the Roman Catholic Church and is about sixteen kilometres away. There is a reliable water system and a sub-post office with telephone services. The National Bank of Commerce is about twelve kilometres away, and many customers patronize it every day.

The weather in Rombo is normally warm and wet. Heavy rains fall twice a year, making the area a wet one almost throughout the year. The rich volcanic soil and good weather conditions make the area suitable for agriculture. The main cash crop, which yields a good income, is coffee. The per capita income of Rondo people is higher than for most other farmers in the country. Food crops include maize, beans, potatoes, and bananas, which is the staple food. Hunger has never hit the area. Generally, the residents are in good health.

Despite the area's agricultural productivity, the youth is mainly engaged in business. Throughout the day, youths are busy moving from one place to another, particularly to the border to sell food crops in exchange for clothes, cooking oil, and cosmetics. Hardly anyone is at home during the mornings. They are either at the market selling their commodities or moving from place to place to sell somewhere else. Businesses like shopkeeping, running restaurants, guesthouses, and importing and exporting commodities are engaged in by locals. Most of the government officers, teachers, policemen, bankers, etc., are from the area, since the educational level of the inhabitants is above primary school level.

Secondary school is the medium level of education for the youths and about one-quarter of them have achieved a higher educational level. It is not common to spot jobless corners in this area. However, in the afternoons, youths are seen in groups having a drink or engaging in social activities. Hardly 10 per cent of the youths are engaged in farming. The majority of them are involved in one or other type of business.

Thus, the socioeconomic status of Keni Aleni village is higher than that of Gairo. The boys have primary and secondary school education, and some had even attended other higher institutions of learning. Their parents' education also ranged from primary school to the graduate level. In their leisure time, the boys in Keni Alleni read magazines, attend discos, and watch video shows. Evidently, boys in the two areas are brought up by their parents in very different home and community settings.

Mkafaida from Keni Aleni tells his story

Mkafaida is 19 years old, the fourthborn to his mother. She is a nurse and his father is graduate, employed as a headmaster in the Christian secondary school. The family lives in a house on their two-acre coffee farm. Today, they have electricity and a telephone service. Since childhood, Mkafaida intended to have a higher education. At primary school he usually was number two, three, four in the class, but at secondary school his performance deteriorated.

> I became very naughty. It was a boarding school. I spent most of my time causing chaos in my class and fighting. I was expelled several times from school and my father had to take me back and force me to apologize to my teachers. My secondary school record was bad. I could no longer go on with school, a thing that I regret today. At the moment, I attend a training school to study electricity. My hobbies are video shows, reading magazines, and going to the disco.

I ask him what he knows about female maturity.

> I am aware that above 10 years girls start showing physical growth like the enlargement of breasts and buttocks. Inside them the reproductive organs also develop and menarche confirms that a girl is able to bear children. Girls mature around 12 years while boys mature around 14 years. From biology class, I came to understand that when a boy matures he is able to cause a pregnancy although I find it hard to understand how this can happen at such an early age. I have seen girls who fall pregnant at less than 20 years suffer a lot. Some die in the course of delivery, or the child dies. Abortions, which cause death, are mostly done for pregnant teenage girls.

> Mature girls are attractive to boys, that is why boys are tempted to start friendships with them. Girls are the major talk of teenage boys. If you see

a group of boys talking or laughing, be assured that girls are among the things they are talking about. They talk about a girl's beauty, which boy is a friend of which girl, who dropped his girlfriend, who has many girl-friends, and who did what to his girlfriend, and such things. Actually, from such talk boys learn a lot about how to win girls and how to be smart and have several girls without causing chaos. Sometimes, your peers may want proof that you have a girlfriend in the form of photos or letters. If you fail to satisfy them, your peers will start to look down on you.

Our activities with girls are letter writing, going to discos or to any public gatherings. Pairing up for school activities matters a lot because this allows you to show your friends who your girl is. Secrecy is very limited among boys. I do not personally like some boys' behaviour towards young girls. Most boys can claim that they have had a sexual relationship with a girl. Some boys change from one girl to another because they believe that by doing so their reputation improves, while in fact the opposite is true. Some boys go to the extent of beating girls and claime that she has insulted him, while in truth it is because she has refused to go out with him. At a later age, when over 16, most boys have a sexual relationship with the girls. Frequently, boys refuse responsibility for the pregnancy they have caused. Having multiple partners, is common and as a result STDs are common too. Once a boy gets an STD, he proudly tells his friends who sometimes congratulate him for having a good number of girls. In some cases, the boy can reveal the name of the girl who infected him and warn the others about her. After treatment, he moves to another girl without fear. STDs to teenage boys are diseases indicating manhood. From peer-group talks I came to understand that most boys do not like to use condoms to avoid STDs, but they do use them for fear of AIDS.

Some girls too behave badly. Some teenage girls have multiple partners and practise pre-marital sex. Most girls want to dress in expensive dresses even when their incomes will not allow this. Instead, they get money from boys or even from married men by befriending them. Some unmarried girls go from one area to another to do business. This is not bad us such, but later they come home with children. This is a clear proof that some girls pretend to be doing business while they are in fact doing something else. A few girls are well behaved. They live with their parents and obey them. They keep single partners and do not go to town without a known purpose. They can be doing business but they don't mix business with love affairs. This is the type of girl who gets married.

I do not like unmarried girls who fall pregnant and have no boy responsible for the pregnancy to marry. I consider such girls to be bad. If she had a stable and well behaved partner then the boy would not let her down. In this community, such a girl will hardly get a man to marry because falling pregnant out-of-wedlock is unacceptable; even the baby has no inheritance in any clan. He cannot own land since he has no paternal parents. We inherit from the father's clan and not mother's. Personally, I would rather advise a girl to use contraceptives rather than to fall pregnant. Contraceptive use is not bad as long as it is under a doctor's prescription so that side-effects are avoided.

Both the boys describe their own development from naive curiosity to undiscriminating desire, and to a greater appreciation of more stable commitments. In the process, they end up using double standards: they used to hunt for girls who were easy prey, and they start to look for the "good girls" who do not roam the streets at night and they dissociate themselves from their female age-mates who fall pregnant in the course of the game. They also testify to the pressures from their peers, and their anxiety about not achieving to the standards of manhood.

The next section relates what I learned from the twenty boys that I interviewed.

How boys learn about sex

In most African tribes, the physical changes associated with maturity are explained during the initiation rites. The boys of Gairo indicated that they passed through initiation ceremonies, but possibly the information they received did not cover all the important issues concerning sexuality. They were mostly taught, it seems, about how to have sex with girls. While they understood the physical and biological changes associated with female maturity, they did not know about periods for safe sex.

Moreover, some believed that a boy of 13 or 14 years was too young to cause pregnancy. Nzala, a 15-year-old Gairo boy, was astonished: "What?, a 13-year-old boy causing pregnancy? I have never heard of such thing. What type of a child would be born? A strange creature (*mdudu*)!" Due to their lack of knowledge about reproduction, the boys associated the growing of a beard with reproduction. They believe that when a boy has grown beard and is over 16, he can impregnate a girl. Boys who had impregnated girls thought that having sex with a mature girl is looking for trouble, because a pregnancy is likely to occur.

The boys received most of their information from their peer-group rather than from elders. Peer-group talk, interpreting proverbs, or dancing styles, observing certain signs, seeing pictures or watching animals are some of the ways teenage boys learn about sex. For example, a teenage boy from Keni Aleni was 8 years old when he heard

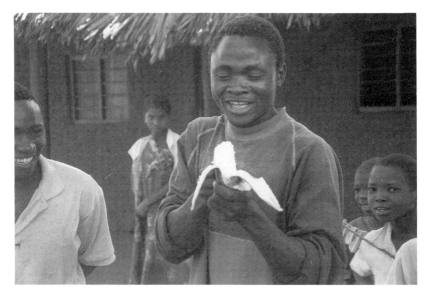

One boy ate a banana in an obsene way, sucking it
and moving it in and out of his mouth, to the laughter
of the other boys.

(Photo Rita Liljeström)

senior boys at school singing a love song: later he learned the meaning
of the song. He also asked his grandfather why roosters bite hens. His
grandfather told him that they were inserting eggs into the hens. Later
he saw cows and goats behaving in the same way. He then concluded
that men and women must do the same thing. His views were
repeated by other teenage boys. The boys' ways of learning about sex
reveal that they are not instructed about manhood and reproduction
as their forebears used to be in traditional African societies.

With modernization and urbanization, initiation rites are dying
out. Boys get more information from peer-groups than from elders.
Both boys and girls are misinformed about or ignorant of
reproductive health issues. They gather information here and there in
the streets. As Kamuzora (1987) and Kassimoto (1985) note, the level
of misinformation or ignorance among youths is appalling.

How does friendship start between boys and girls?

There are various reasons people become friends. Girls and boys do so
through group pressure, the need for status, prestige, attractiveness,
and the need for companionship. In childhood, boys and girls become

friends mainly for companionship. Girls and boys meet at school, at home, at church or water supply areas. They escort each other to distant places, stroll together, share jokes and foodstuffs. Sayi of Gairo narrated his story of how he got his girl. "Personally I started having a girlfriend because all my friends had one. I was 10 years old when I met my girl. I walked with her. I did not approach her and tell her anything. I just used to buy her sweets and drinks."

As boys grow older, the meaning of friendship with girls changes. They are young and would like to practice what they learn from their peers or during initiation ceremonies. Instead of being open they start being furtive: meeting on dark corners at night, in unfinished houses, on farms, outside the village, at bars, local beer shops, guest houses, or at friends homes. While the majority of Gairo boys (nine out of ten) mentioned sex as the major activity during these encounters, the main activities among Keni Aleni friends were going for drinks together, disco as well as traditional dancing, letter writing, group study, and gift giving. Boys feel that they are now mature and it is time to show their manhood. They believe that in order to be recognized by the community as a man, one must have a girlfriend. One is considered smart by talking to her and weak if one is reticent.

The physical changes in girls attracted the boys. Several means are used to show the girl these feelings. These include making frequent jokes with the girl, helping her to solve mathematics problems at school, and boasting to s friend that such and such girl loves him. Sayi of Gairo had a hard time finding a girlfriend. At the age of 10 his peers had girlfriends. Discussion about girls dominated the group. His friends laughed at him, saying he was not handsome and that was why no girls were attracted to him. At the age of 14, he wanted to prove them wrong and show them that he was also a man who could have a girl like them. He approached a girl living in his neighbourhood. Unfortunately he was disappointed. Then one day in his class, a boy snatched a pencil from a girl, and ran away with it. Sayi pursued him and recovered the pencil for the girl. That was the beginning of their friendship.

Boys form strong friendships with girls by buying them presents like sweets, bananas, or sugarcane and by paying special attention to the parents of the girl they love. In considering the problems facing pregnant teenage girls, the boys felt that it was essential for girls to use contraceptives. Boys were strongly against unmarried girls taking contraceptives in normal situations, for fear of the side-effects of the pill. In this case, the boys were sympathetic to the health problems girls might face either by becoming pregnant while still very young or by taking contraceptives without proper supervision. Keni Aleni boys believe that 20 is the proper age for girls to bear children, while Gairo boys consider 17 years to be the appropriate age. Gairo boys' perceptions may be influenced by the traditional views on starting sex at a young age.

Beauty is in the eye of the beholder. To be seen as attractive depends on the preference of the person concerned. Boys indicated that views on the attractiveness of girls varied from one boy to another. Some like a certain girl because of her figure, other like quiet girls. A few boys used their friends to choose a girl for them. These friends conveyed the message to the girls, who would then respond and the relationship would start. Most boys said that if they approach a girl and the girl gives no reply but shows an interest when they talk, they take it for granted that the girl has accepted the proposal.

Male behaviour that is disapproved of

Bad or good behaviour depends on the norms and perceptions of the society concerned. The boys in the two areas indulge in sexual activities. There are some activities which most boys considered to be bad. One form of bad behaviour the boys cited is having multiple partners. However, there were different opinions. The boys who had many girlfriends felt proud of this fact but the other boys, the observers, hated this conduct. Mikureme from Keni Aleni enjoyed having many girlfriends. He said that after he completed his primary school education at the age of 15, he started having sex with a young girl of 12. He bought her presents and the girl accepted him. They met in a dark place and he enjoyed the affair. The sexual act brought him closer to the girl. Notwithstanding this, he did not confine himself to this girl, but continued to play the field with different girls.

Another form of bad behaviour is making false promises to a girl in order to win her. A girl is promised by the boy that they will get married, so she discards all other boyfriends, including serious ones. Later, the girl realizes that the boy has been false. The boy ultimately drops her. Boys also dislike the spreading of information to peers about the girls with whom they have had sexual relations. However, the boy who spreads the information feels proud because he has shown himself to be a man.

They also named other conduct that they disapproved of, such as impregnating girls and then refusing to take responsibility for the pregnancy or convincing girls to perform an abortion, an act which can cause death. Violence and sexual abuse against girls is also condemned. What is viewed as bad sexual conduct was the same for boys from Keni Aleni and from Gairo. It should be remembered that they are all involved in sexual relations, although most of the boys need more guidance on how to practise safe sex and avoid causing problems to for girlfriends.

Good and bad girls

There are three types of girls identified by boys in both areas. There are good girls who stay with their parents and help with household chores. These girls are favoured by all the boys, who appreciate and admire their respectable character. The qualities in girls most liked by boys are helping on the farm, fetching water, and being active in small businesses like selling water and foodstuff. These girls are satisfied with a low income and are not easily cheated by rich men in order to get more money. They have one boyfriend at a time, do not go out for late evening drinks or spend nights in discos, and do not mix business with love.

The other two types are bad girls. There are the promiscuous bad girls who do not move from the village. These girls leave their homes and lodge in rooms somewhere in the area without having a reliable income. They roam the bars at night, drink beer, and do shameful things. These girls cause many marriages to break up because they drink with other women's husbands without wanting to get married. They dress in expensive clothes while their income is low. They do not work on the farms and disrespect their parents.

Then there are girls who move out of the village and go to the big towns on the pretence of looking for employment. Later they return to the village wearing expensive clothes and lavish cosmetics. They normally lie about their places of work. They mention big factories and companies, but they actually sleep with several men for money. These girls later come back home infected with AIDS from which they die. AIDS is associated with the movement of girls to big towns, and the boys condemned such girls.

I noted that although Keni Aleni boys also condemn the idea of promiscuity, they accept the movement of girls from place to place in order to do some business, as long as they do not misbehave. They admire girls who dress well and appear smart. In fact, boys encourage girls to engage in income generating activities but rejected the idea of their having multiple partners.

Proofs of manhood, risks for women

Most people know about those things in which they have an interest and which are likely to happen frequently. Teenage pregnancy is an issue which has been talked about at length by people and institutions. The problems encountered by girls when they become pregnant before the age of 20 has been aired over the radio, by means of pamphlets distributed to the people, and by educational programmes such as seminars and workshops. Do boys have any interest in the problems facing pregnant teenage girls?

I noted that teenage pregnancies were very common in Gairo whereas they were not as common in Keni Aleni. Boys knew the dangers that faced adolescent pregnant girls. Some of the dangers mentioned were anaemia, premature delivery, maternal deaths and child mortality, illegal abortion, and caesarean births. Several examples were cited by Gairo boys of the problems teenage girls faced. This suggests that teenage pregnancies are common.

Mubezi of Gairo cited an example of a girl who died of anaemia and failed to give birth. She died before her relatives could donate blood to her. Anaemic cases were common in Gairo. Cases of caesarean section for teenage girls were frequent. Moreover, premature delivery and three cases in which the girls lost their children during delivery were mentioned. Girls who died during delivery were familiar to the boys. They also knew a case where a teenage girl died when trying to perform an abortion. The instances cited were known to the boys and evidently touched their feelings. The prevalence of teenage pregnancy complications, especially of anaemia leading to maternal death, were corroborated in the medical records of Gairo.

Boys in Keni Aleni also know the problems associated with teenage pregnancies. However, they were able to identify only very few girls who had experienced them. The main issue, as seen by Keni Aleni boys, was that of expulsion of girls from school.

Unmarried pregnant girls

In most African traditional societies, premarital pregnancies were condemned. The patrilineal Wahaya for example, would torture the pregnant girl and she would be left on a desolate island to die. In other tribes, as among the matrilineal Kasai of central Zaire, for example, a girl could only be married after falling pregnant thereby proving her fertility (Kassimoto, 1985:38). Various ethnic groups had different outlooks towards pregnancy. With moderrnisztion and urbanization, I wanted to know how the boys viewed the issue.

They all demonstrated negative attitudes towards unmarried pregnant girls. Even the boys who had fathered babies believed that conception was the girl's mistake. Pregnancy is regarded as some kind of punishment for bad deeds by the girl. However, the boys' outlook towards pregnant girls differed between Gairo and Keni Aleni. In Gairo, half of the ten said they would marry pregnant girls while the others would not. On the other hand, the teenage boys of Gairo who would not accept a pregnant girl, would be particularly unaccepting of a girl who went on to mention several other men as having impregnated her. Such a girl is considered unreliable and unfaithful (*kiruka njia*). The boys' rejection of her in marriage is seen as the penalty for her behaviour in accepting multiple partners. The first pregnancy is seen as the precedent for her having more children by different fathers, none of whom would marry her. Good girls, who fall pregnant get married to the man responsible for the pregnancy. The attitudes of the less accepting Gairo boys remain ambivalent. On the one hand, under certain conditions they would consider marriage to a pregnant girl, but on the other, they fear that she cannot be trusted.

None of the Keni Aleni boys would accept a pregnant girl. They would be ready to take care of the child and the girl only if the girl's behaviour is good. A good girl is one whose life conforms to the behavioural values noted above.

In Keni Aleni, there are few cases of out-of-wedlock pregnancy. An out-of-wedlock mother is considered a curse on the family and is shunned by the community. The unborn child has no future in his/her mother's family's property and can inherit nothing. Such a mother can seldom find a boy to marry. The custom is so entrenched that every member of the community has to observe it. One boy commented: "If a girl claimed that I was responsible, I would deny it because I don't live with her so the child could belong to someone else. If someone else's child joins my family it can be a bad omen for the entire clan. None of my family members would accept that child and its mother. No one in my clan has ever married such a girl and I am not prepared to do so."

Consequently, a girl who falls pregnant out-of-wedlock in Keni Aleni seldom finds a boy to marry. She can normally only get married to an elderly person or widowed man. Her reputation is destroyed in the entire community. If the boy responsible accepts paternity and marries her, his relatives will look down on him as well.

Contraceptives, sexually transmitted diseases and AIDS

All the boys of Gairo and Keni Aleni knew about contraceptives. They got information on them from radio programmes, pamphlets distributed in hospitals, and displays in health clinics and other offices. The use of contraceptives is a way of preventing unplanned pregnancies. The teenage boys' attitudes towards girls using contraceptives differed between Gairo and Keni Aleni boys.

Whereas the teenage boys of Gairo felt it was right for women to choose the type of contraceptives they wanted, because they were the ones who fall pregnant, face pregnancy-related problems, and take care of any children, they strongly object to teenage girls using pills as they are young and do not have children. One respondent, Maleta, was astonished by my question on contraceptives being used by girls. He said, "My fear is these young unmarried girls who go for *vidonge* (pills). What are they after, except bad conduct? I think young girls should not be given pills until they are married."

According to Gairo boys, use of pills by teenage girls means the girl is promiscuous. They also relate the use of contraceptives by girls to some women having no children. The use of condoms by teenage boys is widely accepted. It is surprising that the boys who use girls to satisfy their sexual urges while not wanting them to fall pregnant, do not like the idea of pills. The reason might be the prevailing double standards.

The teenage boys of Keni Aleni accepted the use of contraceptives for all women. They emphasized that all women who need contraceptives should use them under doctor's prescription. Though they accepted girls' use of contraceptives, they did feel that this would encourage premarital relationships. Nevertheless, they felt that it is better to use contraceptives than to have an out-of-wedlock pregnancy. They were of the opinion that contraceptives should be distributed by hospitals or MCH clinics only, to prevent their misuse. Medical shops should not be allowed to sell them.

STDs are expected to occur and are seen as a sign of teenagers being active and having several partners. They are common among the boys and they said that it showed manhood. The teenage boys did not view STDs as something abnormal. Rather they viewed contraction of STD by a boy as normal. Boys go with girls and STDs are among the expected consequences: Every work has its price.

The most common disease in the two areas is gonorrhoea. It is easily transmitted and easily cured. Everybody expect to contract this disease at one time or an other. A boy who contracts the disease goes to the medical shop and buys a dose of ampicillin. Boys do not feel ashamed of about the disease and they talk about it to their peers. One major requirement for getting cured is money to buy the medicine. After being cured, the boys try to avoid the last girl they had sex with and they warn their friends to avoid her. They show no concern for the girls' health.

Syphilis is rare in the two areas. The boys were aware that syphilis is dangerous and causes pimples and damages the boy's sexual parts.

All the teenage boys of the two areas are aware that AIDS has no cure and that a common way of spreading it is through sex. They get information concerning the disease from various sources: in schools, churches, community centres, hospitals and other places. Information is aired over the radio and it is disseminated by anti-AIDS campaigners who go from one place to another conducting awareness seminars and showing films. The boys fear AIDS. A group of educated people had visited Gairo and shown them films on the AIDS situation in Bukoba.

The campaigners advised the teenager boys to have sex with only one partner. However, the teenage boys admitted that their sexual conduct has not changed. They fear that in a few years to come girls and boys from the two areas will be afflicted by the disease if their behaviour does not change. Some of them believe in using condoms as a solution, but admitted that they were not using them because they feel uncomfortable.

They believe that AIDS is a townspeople's disease since no AIDS case has originated in their home areas. They claim that victims contracted it in the big towns. Ndelekio of Keni Aleni stated, "We call it '*umeme*' (electricity), slim or the killer. Many people contract it in the big towns and they are brought here to die and get buried in their home village. None has contracted it in our area."

Some comments

My point of departure was to explore teenage boys' views on sexuality, girls, and pregnancies in two communities which differed in several ways:

Gairo village	*Keni Aleni village*
permissive matrilineal Kaguru	strict patrilineal Chagga
people are poor and ill educated	people are well off and well educated
no schools above primary level	secondary and technical schools
outsiders occupy public offices	local elite occupies public offices
rest place for trucks and lorries	lively border trade

The primary school leavers in Gairo search for occasional jobs and a chance to earn some income, while the Keni Aleni boys have access to non-farming activities in the transborder trade. While unemployed Gairo boys gather on the street corners, *kijiweni*, the Keni Aleni boys spend time by reading magazines and watching videos. Do such differences have any bearing on how the boys view sexual matters?

Basically, the boys have more things in common than differences. The differences are more a question of degree than of kind. Keni Aleni boys are stricter in their personal rejection of unmarried pregnant girls for marriage than Gairo boys. This is out of the question in Keni Aleni, whereas half the Gairo boys are willing to marry a single mother, and the other half feels ambivalent, yet willing to accept such a wife under certain conditions.

On the other hand, the Keni Alleni boys are more willing to accept that teenage girls avoid pregnancies by using contraceptives than are the Gairo boys. The Keni Aleni boys also support the income earning activities of girls, even if this means that the girls stay away from home, provided that the girls do not mix business with love affairs. Moreover, the Keni Alleni boys seem to indulge in more varied activities with their girlfriends than the Gairo boys do. The latter appear more interested in just having sex.

My study cannot differentiate between the impact of Kaguru respectively Chagga customs, and the socioeconomic gap between the two villages.

One can discern a psychosocial process in the boys' attitudes towards girls. They start being curious and look for companions. They become more sexually involved and indiscriminate, and later on the social and moral qualities of the girls come to the forefront, regrettably often in a judgmental and hostile way. To be fair, some boys also distance themselves from crude behaviour by other boys. On the positive side, this conduct bears witness to increasing awareness about valid standards for relationships between men and women.

On the other hand, there are more muddy waters than the boys admit, contradictions and double standards. Commonly, having sex with a girl or girls is viewed as a measure of manhood. The girls appear as a means to that end. The boys testify about peer-group pressures leading to having a girlfriend, and to the constant pre-occupation with girls. Even a contracted STDs are regarded as proof of manhood.

The girlfriends expose themselves to great risks: they risk their reputation, education, chances to a good marriage, health, and even their lives. The condemnatory attitudes of their male age-mates, who mostly go free, need to be seriously addressed. The damaging separation of men's and women's sexual interests has to be bridged by communication and by understanding the mutuality of the risks and opportunities.

References

Kassimoto, T.J., 1985, "Attitudes of Parents, Students, Ex-pregnant schoolgirls, and Administrators on the Expulsion of Pregnant Girls from Schools". Unpublished M.A. dissertation. University of Dar es Salaam.

Kamuzora, C.L., 1987, "Adolescent Sexuality Consequences, knowledge and Practice of Contraception and Associated Factors". University of Dar es Salaam. Mimeo.

Chapter 7
Maintenance and Care in Law and Practice

Magdalena K. Rwebangira

We love children

When young children are dumped in pit latrines or left by the roadside to die by their mothers, we condemn them. Likewise, when
fathers expel their pregnant unmarried daughters from their homes,
we condemn them. Indeed, we also blame primary, secondary, and
some vocational schools for discontinuing the education of women
who fall pregnant during the course of their educational programmes.
Officially, most communities, particularly African, regard children as
sacred, not only as gifts from God to be cherished but also as insur-
ance in old age and an investment in the future of the community. The
communities, as well as the state through its law enforcers, have been
eager to punish those who commit criminal acts and try to end the life
of an infant.

I set out to assess the position of unmarried mothers. My interest
arose from a previous study in which I explored the situation of pregnant teenage girls and the legal aspect of contraception, abortion, and
infanticide (Rwebangira, 1992a). This time, my aim is to investigate
the care of children born out-of-wedlock. To this end I have identified
five specific issues I want to highlight:

- Who actually cares for children?;
- Who has custody of or access to the illegitimate child?;
- The sources of monetary settlements for the infants' needs;
- The institutional support the mother and her kin receive through
  court orders, official instructions, counselling service(s), advice,
  etc. and if the same has been useful; and
- Whether the mother has subsequently married and has had to
  make changes in the care arrangements?

In this chapter, unless otherwise explained, custody means the right
and duty to care for and exercise control over the child and its wel-

fare. Access means the non-custodial parent's freedom to communicate with or visit a child. Guardian means a person having charge of an infant of which he or she is not the parent. While the natural father is the biological father or the husband of the mother of a child born in wedlock, the putative father is the alleged or reputed father of a child born out-of-wedlock.

The legal position

The legal system of Tanzania is governed by a plural regime. There is the general law composed of laws received from England,[1] those enacted by the British colonial government before independence, as well as those passed by the postindependence parliament. Another system of law is customary law which has been codified as it applies to patrilineal communities only. These make up 80 per cent of the country's diverse population. The other 20 per cent are traditionally matrilineal and have their own customary law (James and Fimbo, 1973). However, many people still use variations of customary law as it applies to their locality. It is this pluralism which successive governments have attempted (or failed) to deal with in order to progressively achieve legal uniformity. For example, the *Law of Marriage Act (LMA)* 1971 provides that customary and Islamic laws shall not apply to matters provided for in the *LMA*.[2]

Application of Laws

The Customary Law Declaration Order 1963 provides that "all children born in wedlock belong to the father (Rule 175). Whereas those born out-of-wedlock are designated to belong to the maternal family unless legitimized by their father. They are the responsibility of the maternal grandfather (Rule 178). The father of an illegitimate child can legitimize it by payment of 100 shillings to the girl's father or by marrying

---

[1] See the Reception Clause which applied English law to Tanzania under the Tanganyika Order in Council 1920 proclaimed on 22 July 1920. The relevant article stated that jurisdiction should be exercised in conformity with the common law, the doctrines of equity, and the statutes of general application in force in England at the time of passing the order. This general Reception Clause is reenacted with a few minor modifications by the *Judicature and Application of Laws Ordinance*, Cap. 453, 1961.

[2] See section 9(3A) of the *Judicature and Application of Laws Ordinance*, Cap. 453, as amened by the *Law of Marriage Act* 1971, Second Schedule.

the mother of the child (Rule 181(a) and (b)). The domicile of the child is to be arranged by both mother and father and the court can intervene if they fail to agree.

Technically this law is not applicable to the matrilineal communities of the country. Nonetheless, research among these communities has shown that when unwed mothers and other guardians of children born out-of-wedlock have sought maintenance from the children's natural fathers as provided by the *Law of Marriage Act*, 1971 (S. 129–30), the said fathers have claimed custody of the children. Ironically, as with the case of divorcing mothers, the courts have been inclined to grant custody of the children to their fathers when it was convenient for the latter (Rwebangira, 1991).

The Adoption Ordinance, Cap. 335

The *Adoption Ordinance* gives due significance to actual custody of the infant and to the people liable to contribute to the maintenance of the child. Thus, in an application for adoption of infants, the law requires that the following people must be served with a copy of the petition: the parent or parents, the guardian or guardians, and *the person or persons having the actual custody of the infant* as well as *the persons liable to contribute to the support of the infant* (see Rules of Court, G.N. 1942, No. 321, Vol. V, pp. 237–45). In a petition for adoption, both the natural father and the mother are giving precedence in consenting to the adoption. The "father" in relation to an illegitimate infant, is defined to mean the natural father (S. 2(1)). This law is significant for the mothers of children born out-of-wedlock, because it provides another means of integrating such children into a nuclear family under the general law.

Adoption is a process whereby a court makes an order creating new parents for the child. Adoption law in Tanzania is governed by the *Adoption Ordinance*, Cap. 335. It owes its legal history to the English *Adoption of Children's Act* of 1926, introduced into Tanzania in 1942, as the *Adoption of Infants' Ordinance* and mildly amended in 1953 and 1968. Under this law, adults wishing to adopt an infant have to apply to the High Court. The applicant has to be at least 25 years of age and at least 21 years older than the child, unless he/she is a relative or parent of the child, in which case such age requirements are dispensed with.

The *Adoption Order* vests the adopter with all parental rights and responsibilities relating to the child. Likewise, natural parents lose corresponding parental rights and are relieved of their parental responsibilities. Moreover, the child is also deprived of the right to inherit from its natural parents when they die.

A child born out-of-wedlock can be adopted. The application can be made by the natural parent jointly with a spouse if such parent is married. If the application is made jointly and the court grants the adoption order, both husband and wife would have equal rights and responsibilities towards the child as if the child had been born in wedlock. Nonetheless, where only one spouse applies for adoption, the law requires that the other spouse should consent to the application and the implied responsibility that goes with the new relationship that is being sought.

Would this work well in patrilineal communities, where a child is considered to belong to its father's lineage and not a woman's? In such communities, the mother's husband may not give his consent to his wife's adoption of her illegitimate child for many reasons, including fear of assuming responsibility and family disapproval. Furthermore, acceptance of the child into the family may be problematic, given the customary procedures and rituals associated with the birth of a child in many traditional communities. An illegitimate child brought into a marriage would still be seen as outside blood by the man's kin, irrespective of legal niceties such as an adoption order.

The findings of a study in remote rural areas of Kagera bears this impression out. The study, conducted in Tanzania in 1985, found that Tanzanians of African descent rarely apply for adoption orders. Applicant stepparents were European husbands and African wives, who were the mothers of the adopted children. The next group was of Asiatic origin (often migrating or living abroad). Indigenous African couples did not feature in these cases at all (Rwezaura and Wanitzek, 1988).

The Affiliation Ordinance

The Affiliation Ordinance is intended to provide for the maintenance of illegitimate children. On application, within the prescribed time, by a pregnant woman or a woman who has delivered a child, the court has the power to summon before it the putative father and, if satisfied that such man is the father of the infant, make an order for the maintenance of the child by the such putative father (Ss. 3, 4, 5). Whereas under customary law, weight is placed on the father's word of honour to accept or dispute paternity, the *Affiliation Ordinance* puts full weight on the mother's word. Rwezaura notes that the assumption behind customary law seems to be that it is prestigious for a man to father a child such that he would dare not deny it if it were true (Rwezaura, 1986–7). Under the *Affiliation Ordinance*, once a pregnant or unwed mother names any man as the father of her child, the onus of proving that such allegation is false shifts to the father. He can only succeed in discharging it by proving that he did not have sexual intercourse with the woman concerned, or that by time lapse or some other reason he could not possibly be the father of the child concerned.[3]

Upon the making of an adoption order in respect of an illegitimate child under the *Affiliation Ordinance*, such child's father's obligation for maintenance ceases to have any effect (S. 13(1)) except where such order is made in favour of an unmarried mother of such child, in which case the father shall continue to be responsible for the child's maintenance. Moreover, such father's responsibility for maintenance also ceases if and when such mother remarries (S. 13(2)). It has been said that such a law is unfair to both the welfare of the mother and the child for two reasons. One is that it predisposes the mother to remain unmarried in her prime, when she is otherwise most likely to get married. Second, it prejudices the child for its mother's lawful action and her exercise of the human right to form a family (Rwebangira, 1991, 1995).

The Law of Marriage Act 1971

This is the main law providing for the rights of women in relation to marriage and parental rights over their children. It does not make a distinction between children born out-of-wedlock and those born in wedlock. Moreover, it provides that where a marriage between parents has been declared a nullity or is annulled by the court, the child born of that union shall be presumed legitimate and, in the absence of agreement or an order of court to the contrary, the mother will be entitled to the custody of the infant child of such union (S. 128).

---

[3] See section 3 and 5 of the *Affiliation Ordinance*, 1949, Cap. 278.

A man has the duty to maintain his infant by providing it with accommodation, clothing, food, and, education, whether such child is in his custody or not, unless there is an agreement or a court order to the contrary. The amount involved in discharging this duty depends on the man's means and his station in life. A father can discharge the duty of maintenance by paying in cash (S. 129(1)). A mother does not carry such corresponding duty for maintenance or contribution to it unless the child(ren)'s father is dead or his whereabouts are unknown or, for some other reason, he is unable to maintain them (S. 129(2)) under certain circumstances (S. 130(1)). A court has corresponding power to order a woman to discharge the duty of maintenance or contribution if such court is satisfied that she has the means to do so (S. 130(2)).

The legal principle governing maintenance as stipulated in sections 129–130 of the *LMA* places the duty on the father to maintain his children by providing them with accommodation, clothing, food, and education whether or not they are in his custody. When it comes to children born out-of-wedlock, the starting point is the *Affiliation Ordinance*, Cap. 278. The amount payable per child per month in law is 100 shillings only, which is grossly insufficient. The *Ordinance* has not been amended since 1964 and has long been overtaken by inflation. When parties have ended up in court, the courts have justifiably ordered higher amounts on several occasions, depending on father's financial ability. Yet maintenance awards are hardly ever sufficient to cover the child's needs, let alone the administrative nightmare of processing its collection. The problem is compounded by the fact that the court can only compute the quantum of maintenance payable from the father's proven wages or general income. Since most people's "official" income is low, maintenance orders are generally low.

Consequently, most single women with young children, irrespective of whether maintenance is sought and awarded or not, live in abject poverty, especially in urban and periurban areas where the subsistence economy is nonexistent. They become a further burden on their relatives who have to support them and their children. In addition to the inadequacy of maintenance rates, maintenance tends to be paid irregularly and the collection process becomes a nightmare for women. Maintenance orders are discharged on the occurrence of one of two things. One is the remarriage of the mother. The other is the resumption of cohabitation by a mother who has lived separately from her husband.

As already noted, this is grossly unfair to the child's welfare and also to the mother. It punishes the child for its mother's lawful act and the exercise of her human right to form a family. It also prejudices the mother's marital status for life for she has to remain single to obtain maintenance for the child born out-of-wedlock, or carry the child as a burden into another marriage or send it away to generous relatives, if any.

The Penal Code, Cap. 16

Care and maintenance of children are considered significant enough to merit penal sanctions. Under section 166 of the *Penal Code*, any parent, guardian, or other person having lawful care of a child under 14 years who is able to maintain such child but who wilfully and without reasonable cause deserts or leaves such child without means or support, is guilty of an offence. Likewise, persons who neglect to provide sufficient food, clothing, bedding, and other necessities for such child in a way that would adversely affect the health of such child are guilty of an offence (S. 167).

These provisions were successfully invoked by the former minister for home affairs, Mr. Augustine Lyatonga Mrema, in the early 1990s, when he used the powers of the state to pin down runaway fathers to pay for the maintenance of both their legitimate and illegitimate children.

Legal history and the welfare of the child

The distinction between custody rights of married and unmarried mothers in the law in Tanzania is a legacy of the *Bastardy Laws* in English law dating back to the Victorian era (Rwezaura, 1985). Under the *Bastardy Laws* responsibility for children born to unwed mothers fell solely on their mothers. In practice, this includes guardianship, custody, and maintenance. This also meant that such children did not have inheritance rights in their father's estates (Smart and Sevenhuijsen, 1989). In Britain (and other Western countries generally) this position of sole custody enjoyed by unwed mothers was to acquire political significance in the twentieth century. The mothers of illegitimate children did not have to tolerate bad relationships in order to stay with their children or maintain access. Both custody and access were theirs as a matter of right. It was argued by middle-class married women that unwed mothers had far more rights than they, the "proper" mothers. It was the evolution of the principle of "the best interests of the child" and a subsequent shift in judicial policy that mitigated this situation for married mothers.

The history of the principle of the paramountcy of the interests or welfare of the child, as it is sometimes called, dates back to British law, specifically under the *Guardianship of Infants Act* 1925 (Section 1(b), which provided that:

> Where in any proceedings before any court ...

> (b) the administration of any property belonging to or held in trust for a minor, or the application of the income thereof, is in question, the court in deciding that question, shall regard the welfare of the minor as the first and paramount consideration and shall not take into consideration whether from any other point of view the claim of the father in respect of such customary, upbringing, administration or application is superior to that of the mother, or the claim of the mother to be superior to that of the father.[4]

The social context in which this legislation was born was one where the husband had absolute rights over all the children born to his wife. Mothers who left their marriages were punished by separation from their children.[5] Many a mother was obliged to tolerate a bad marriage for fear of this separation.[6] Feminists finally succeeded in getting the law reformed to allow women who had taken criminal proceedings against violent husbands to live apart from the latter and take their children of up to 7 years of age.[7] These developments in guardianship were the results of the combined efforts of the feminists and the effect of sociologists' and psychologists' teachings on the significance of mother-child bonding in the child's tender years of development and growth. Thus, the doctrine of tender years, preceded the principle of the paramountcy of the interests of the child. However, it was not to have a profound effect on custody battles until 1970.

By 1969, family ideology and social values had changed, allowing for more interventionist interpretation by the courts. In the case of *J v.*

---

[4] Now the Guardianship of Minors Act 1971.

[5] See Norton, C., 1982, *Caroline Norton's Defence.* Chicago: Academy of Chicago.

[6] Jahled Brenton, 1828, during debates in the House of Lords on reforms to guardianship laws, quoted in Penchbeck I. and M. Hewitt, 1973, *Children in English Society*, Vol. II, pp. 374. London: Routledge & Kegan Paul.

[7] *Matrimonial Causes Act* 1978.

C (1970) the principle of best interests of the child was echoed by the court which held that "custody, access, education or upbringing must be decided on the welfare of the child whether the adults before the court are parents or non-parents".[8]

The father's absolute rights at common law and the punishment of matrimonial guilt, which in practice allowed the presumed guilty party to be punished by deprivation of reliefs like custody, coexisted with the principle of best interests of the child at that time. Thus, in the case of *J v. V* the best interest of the child was applied to deny custody to natural, well-meaning, but incapable parents. This came close to resolving a controversy that had occupied the courts in the 1960s, namely, how far they should go in punishing the guilty parent and, secondly, the weight to be placed on the presumption that, as a general rule, it was better for young children to be brought up by their mothers. There was also the third issue-of-justice claim, whereby the spouse wronged by the other was to be considered more favourably in determining custody.[9] Frequently, it was the adulterous mother who sought custody of an issue of marriage.[10] To balance the interests of the child and justice claims, if both parents fared equally on other points except the misbehaviour, the innocent would be considered more suitable for a custody award. However, by 1977, following the judgment in the case of *J v. C* the Court of Appeal repeatedly held that to balance the welfare of the child against the wishes of an impeachable parent or the justice of the case as between the parties was no longer to be regarded as good law.[11] As a result of this change in judicial policy, an adulterous mother was awarded custody in the case of *Re. K*.[12] In that case the validity of justice claims was put into doubt.

Thus the stage was finally set for determinations based on the paramountcy of the welfare/interest of the child on the break-up of marriage, and devoid of moral judgments on the parents' behaviour

---

[8] Quoted in S. Maidement, 1984, *Child Custody and Divorce*. London: Croom Helm, p. 14.

[9] See Lord Denning in *Re. L* (1962), where he held that "... whilst the welfare of the children is the first and paramount consideration, the claims of justice cannot be overlooked."

[10] See *Re. L* (1962) above.

[11] Compare with Tanzania's *Customary Law Declaration Order* 1963, G.N. No. 279/63, Rule 125.

[12] The position in Britain was not protected by statute until 1975 under the *Common Law Act*.

towards each other. At least presumed guilt was no longer a bar to custody in law. In fact, mothers came to be given custody almost routinely.

As noted earlier on, this was not the case with unwed mothers, whose problem was to obtain assistance, if any, from the natural fathers of their children. In Britain, many of these mothers were poor and had to put their children and themselves in workhouses to survive. This was the basis for the enactment of the *Affiliation Ordinance* in Britain.[13] It is this legal history which was imported into Tanzania in 1949 when the *Affiliation Ordinance* was passed as law, and in 1971 when the principle of the best interests of the child was incorporated in the *Law of Marriage Act*.

Gradually, this historical transplant developed into a visible challenge to patriarchal power, particularly in view of the increasing trend towards non-marital living arrangements. It was feared and still is that more women might opt for autonomous motherhood (Smart, 1989). In Western countries, this fear and the growing need for maintenance of children has given rise to a backlash from fathers against what is seen as court favouritism towards women in custody cases. These men have advocated joint custody and are reluctant to pay maintenance if the mother has sole custody.

Literature is scanty on the subject in Tanzania. There is some information about street children and an indication that children born out-of-wedlock and into broken families form the bulk of the children roaming our streets as beggars. Moreover, other factors such as violence in the home and poverty, contribute to this phenomenon. Mongulla, in his paper titled, "Children under Especially Difficult Circumstances in Tanzania: The Case of Street Children" (1991), cites the circumstances giving rise to street children as being disintegrating family values, single motherhood, unemployment of fathers, low salaries, alcoholism, extra-large families leading sometimes to relegation of children to uncles, brothers, or sisters. Mwakanjala (1993), on the other hand, points out that the hypothesis that most street children are born out-of-wedlock is not true. In his study, only 4 per cent of all the children he interviewed did not have a "proper" family background; that is, they could not tell the whereabouts of their parents. Hence, he concluded that the extended family system was

---

[13] One notes the contradiction in values in the same society between children that nobody wants and those that parents, relatives and institutions are fighting for.

still intact in Tanzania and that children born out-of-wedlock are easily adopted into the extended family circle.

The literature emphasizes the need to understand how far child-care and the maintenance of children born out-of-wedlock may be contributing to the teenage problem in Tanzania, if at all, and the opportunity cost paid by the children's mothers. How much do we know about what out-of-wedlock mothers have to give up in order to bring up their children properly?

In Tanzania, before the enactment of the *LMA* 1971, various personal laws applied to matters of marriage and custody. The legal consideration relating to custody of infant children is stipulated in S. 125 of *LMA*, which holds in effect that the court has power to grant custody to either the mother or the father or any other relative of the infant or any association the objects of which include child welfare. In making this decision, the paramount consideration is to be the welfare of the infant and subject to this, the court shall have regard to both the wishes of the parents and to the wishes of the infant, where he or she is of an age to express an independent opinion (Ss. 2(a)(b)). Furthermore, there is a rebuttable presumption that it is for the good of an infant below the age of 7 years to be with her/his mother, but in deciding whether this presumption applies to the facts of any particular case, the court shall have regard to the undesirability of disturbing the life of an infant by changes of custody (S. 3). Finally, the court is not bound to place all children (of a marriage) under the custody of the same person but shall consider the welfare of each independently (S. 4).

This law does not distinguish between legitimate and illegitimate children. This distinction is made under the *Customary Law Declaration Order (CLDO)* 1963, as we noted earlier.

However, access is dealt with without distinction between married and unmarried women under S. 126 *LMA*, which provides, among other things, the conditions of custody and access to the child by the non-custodial parent.

A study of maintenance in Botswana concluded that single mothers and their children constitute the vast majority of the poor vulnerable groups.[14] Similar studies in Swaziland and Lesotho found that women are afraid of claiming maintenance for fear of losing custody

---

[14] Botswana, 1991, Preliminary Research Report, Women and Law in Southern Africa (WLSA).

of their children or else of harm befalling them through witchcraft.[15]
Similar trends can be found in Tanzania. This raises the question of
what then happens to these children? Recent interviews with street
children in Dar es Salaam indicate that most of them are either from
broken families or have run away from "mistreatment" at home or
from other domestic problems (Rwebangira, 1991). Some of their
mothers may have been teenagers when they were born! Whose legal
responsibility are they and how does this affect their mothers?

The law rarely gives holistic answers to concrete social problems.
Often it selectively acknowledges the existence of some situations
while maintaining silence on others. It is because of this fragmentation
of life, that some scholars of feminist jurisprudence call for a beyond-
law approach (Dahl, 1987; Smart, 1989).

Little study seems to have been undertaken on the issue of custody and access to children born out-of-wedlock to teenage mothers in
Tanzania. However, some work has been done on these aspects in respect of married parents. In that regard, both the law and the courts
have been criticized for overemphasizing factors which favour fathers
in custody disputes (Rwebangira, 1988, 1991). Access to children of
divorces has been cited as particularly problematic when the infant is
in the care of an ex-husband who has subsequently remarried. But
custody with a mother, be she married or not, has been singled out as
source of post-divorce conflict and intrusion by the former husband,
although a few success stories have also been noted (Rwebangira,
1991). In feminist jurisprudence, "access" is seen as joint custody and
objected to on two accounts. One is that it would simply extend men's
power over women without necessarily protecting the interest of the
children. Secondly, that children need to be cared for on a day-to-date
basis and it is mothers who provide this primary care (Smart and
Sevenhuijsen, 1989). Both these factors are likely to be overshadowed
in the contest for parental rights (Freeman, 1984). In Tanzania, this de-
bate has yet to begin. Probably due to the lack of formal social benefits
and the economic powerlessness of the large majority of mothers
compared to men, courts tend to place higher value on the parent who
can provide better economic support (Rwebangira, 1992b). Joint custody, therefore, is seen as the best of both worlds.

---

[15] Swaziland and Lesotho, 1991, National Research Reports, Women and Law in
Southern Africa (WLSA).

As for teenage mothers who are virtually children themselves, what parental rights do they want and deserve in the care of their children? In the absence of social welfare benefits such as child allowances and unemployment benefits, what rights or obligations do mothers have towards their children? Issues of competing rights between children and women are becoming an increasing challenge for feminism and women's law in particular. Teenage motherhood out-of-wedlock could be a further delicate test. A number of chapters in the present study illustrate the dilemmas of such young mothers, as they choose between their own future and that of their children.

There are other studies, as well. Salma Moulid's on the subject in Tanzania, entitled "The Issue of Custody and Maintenance of Children Born-Out-of-Wedlock"[16] looks into the practices of religious institutions, among other things. She found that the Roman Catholic denomination was not institutionally geared towards custody or maintenance of children affected by separation or divorce, let alone those born out-of-wedlock. She explained the reasons as being that the three situations are either unacceptable or frowned on in the church's doctrines. In principle, the situation was found to be the same in the Lutheran church. However, where the couple was experiencing difficulties leading to unbearable hardship, the two churches preferred that the children be left with the mother if the couple separated.

The conciliation boards operating under the auspices of these two religious institutions, however, admitted that they ask the father to contribute to the maintenance of such child(ren) according to his ability. However, children born out-of-wedlock or of an adulterous relationship do not receive such attention. She noted that custody and maintenance cases were common in social welfare offices. The offices help the parties to reach an amicable settlement regardless of whether or not the relationship between the parents is legal or even moral. It was against that background that the present study set out to learn more about the caring of children born to teenage mothers out-of-wedlock, and about emerging trends in this area.

Research areas and methods

The study was conducted in the Coast and Kagera regions respectively. Kibaha, Bunju, and Bagamoyo were covered in the coast region

---

[16] 3rd year Compulsory Research Paper.

while Kishanje and Buganguzi wards of Bukoba and Muleba districts respectively were covered in Kagera region. The distribution of respondents is as follows:

Coast region			*Kagera region*		
	fathers	mothers		fathers	mothers
Kibaha	17	20	Kishanje ward, Bukoba	0	1
Bunju	9	11	Buganguzi ward, Muleba district)	1	9

In total, 66 respondents participated in the general survey. Furthermore, five people were selected for case studies in Kibaha, Bunju, and Buganguzi each respectively.

The timeframe was between January 1993 and July 1995. These regions were selected primarily for comparative purposes. The methods I employed include archival research, interviews, home visits, life histories, and focus group discussions. The general pattern proceeded from the gathering of general information to individual interviews, home visits, and dissemination or validation workshops.

The research was preceded by a pilot study in 1993. Except in Kishanje ward,[17] the study was concluded by a workshop in the form of a focus group discussion with between twenty and twenty-five participants. These workshops were attended by selected teenage girls, parents of teenage girls, former teenage mothers, religious leaders, health workers, magistrates, social welfare officers, and related workers. The participants identified themes and the meeting split into three discussion groups. The separate groups were composed of adult women, men, and teenage mothers (former and present) respectively. The groups deliberated on the themes and made recommendations which were reported back to the plenary. It was at the plenary presentation that gender contestation came into sharp relief. A combination of these methods enabled me to collect relevant information for my research.

Coast region

The inhabitants of the Coast region are traditionally matrilineal. The affiliation of children among them is with maternal uncles. Premarital

---

[17] There was a funeral in the village.

sex is less restrictive compared to patrilineal societies. Kibaha and Bagamoyo districts are said to be ethnically diverse. Kibaha district houses the regional headquarters for the Coast region. Its location is adjacent to the main highway, the Morogoro road, leading to Dar es Salaam. Its population, therefore, consists of many people not indigenous to the district.

Bagamoyo on the other hand is to the south of the city, out of the way, and bordering on the Indian Ocean. The literature indicates that despite its proximity to the doorway of the country (the Indian Ocean); and its early contact with foreign traders and conversion to Islam, the inhabitants of Bagamoyo have remained traditional at heart, more or less committed to their traditional ways of life (Swantz, 1985). Although my study could not be completed in Bagamoyo due to floods which washed away the bridges at Mpiji and Chalinze, the results in the neighbouring ward of Bunju do reveal this tendency.[18]

Kibaha

Kibaha is one of the districts making up the Coast region. It is home to the regional headquarters. The social welfare office in Kibaha technically serves both Kibaha and Bagamoyo districts but operates out of Kibaha because of transportation and other logistical difficulties, and is, therefore, more accessible to Kibaha residents. Furthermore, there is no social welfare office in Bagamoyo and the regional office does its work there through the community development office.

Caring for children born out-of-wedlock

There were nine affiliation cases in 1990, nine in 1991, and nineteen in 1993. Although putative fathers were identified in all cases in 1990 and 1991 and in eighteen out of nineteen in 1993, none of these fathers subsequently married the mothers of their children. In these thirty-seven cases, thirteen mothers were cohabiting with the fathers of the children either regularly or on a temporary basis, although they continued to collect maintenance payments from the social welfare office.

---

[18] The results were validated and disseminated in the neighbouring ward of Bunju, 26 kilometres from the city centre, although technically in Dar es Salaam region. The inhabitants are of the same ethnic origin (Wakwere, Wangindo, Wazaramo, etc.) as those who live in Bagamoyo.

Only two cases had been referred to court. In eleven of the cases, the fathers were only contributing towards the maintenance of the children and wanted nothing to do with the mother. Four cases were unknown, as the women ceased to use the services of the social welfare office. The nature of maintenance contributions by fathers differed, but some were in kind and not monetary. There were only two cases where the father absolutely refused to have anything to do with the child.

I define care to include provision of shelter, clothes, and food, as well as bathing, washing, feeding, and school fees and materials for those children who are old enough to go to school. In Kibaha, in two-thirds of the cases some care was provided by the teenage mothers, in one-half by mostly maternal grandparents and occasionally other relatives, and only in one-quarter of the cases was care provided by the putative fathers.

Regarding crucial assistance from the teenage mothers' relatives such as delivery, food, medical care, and physical childhandling chores, mothers and sisters were reported to be particularly helpful, especially in providing food and childcare. In about one-third of the examples the relatives could not help because they lived far from the teenage mothers.

Provision of material needs such as clothing was mainly by mothers of the children in two-thirds of the cases. Grandparents met this need in five cases only out of twenty. Other sources of clothing materials are a combination of parents and aunts.

Half the children (ten) get food from their mothers, and grandparents provide food to four children. Other suppliers of food included an aunt, mother and sister, mother and parents, mother and father, and father alone.

As to helping the child keep clean, fifteen teenage mothers washed their children whereas four children were assisted by their grandparents. An aunt provided this service to only one child. As for other services, these were provided by mothers in three-quarters of the cases while grandparents helped in the rest.

Meeting the cost of buying soap is done by the mothers of all the children. As before, next are the grandparents, who helped to provide soap to three children. The mother and father provided soap jointly in two cases.

The teenage mothers were asked about meeting the cost f buying pencils, exercise books, school fees, and uniforms. This question was relevant in a few cases, in all of which the costs were being met by mothers themselves. In seventeen cases, there was no response probably because the children were still too young to go to school.

Profile of putative fathers

Seventeen putative fathers were also interviewed in Kibaha. The biggest single group (five out of seventeen) were 30 years of age. Twenty-eight years is the average age for the putative fathers. Nine of the seventeen putative fathers were formally employed while five were engaged in business. Other occupations were welding and peasant farming coupled with petty business.

Table 1. *Caring for the children response by 9 mothers in Muleba*

	Mother	Father	G.father	G.mother	Parents	Total
Housing	1	-	2	6	-	9
Clothing	1	-	2	6	-	9
Food *						9
Washing clothes	4	-	5	-	-	9
Buying soap	3	-	1	5	-	9
School needs	-	-	1	2	-	3
Bathing	4	-	5	-	-	9

* All farming and in one case both farming and buying

Table 2. *Caring for children in Bunju: Responses by 9 fathers*

	Mother	Father	Parents	No answer	Brother	Total
Housing	1 m+f	5	-	-	-	9
Clothing	-	6	-	2	1	9
Food	-	6	-	2	1	9
Washing clothes	-	7	-	2	-	9
Buying soap	-	8	-	1	-	9
School needs	-	4	-	5	(helped 1)	9
Bathing	-	3	-	6	-	9
Financial help	1	-	3	5	-	9

According to the summary of responses shown in Table 1 above, the fathers do very little to care for the children in Buganguzi, compared to the mothers and grandparents. But the fathers in Bunju consider that they provide most needs of the children while the mothers provide almost nothing.

Table 3. *Caring for children in Kibaha: Response by 17 fathers*

	Mother	Father	Jointly	Grand	Brother	Uncle	Total
Housing	-	10	-	-	1	1	12
Clothing	1	11	-	-	-	-	12
Food	6	9	2	-	-	-	17
Washing clothes	7	5	-	5	-	-	17
Buying soap		12(70%)	-	-	-	-	12
Bathing	4	5	3	-	-	-	12
School needs	-	4	-	-	-	-	17
General care	1	11	plus	seven	parents	jointly	19

In Table 3, although Kibaha fathers credit themselves for providing for their out-of-wedlock children more than did the mothers, there was greater acknowledgement of the teenage mothers' contribution to providing the children with necessities. This may be due to the fact that most of the mothers in Kibaha had some income of their own.

When asked who provides food for the children, nine fathers said they did so themselves. Food was said to be provided jointly by the mother and father in two cases only. The putative fathers admitted that the mothers were the sole providers of food for the children in six cases. According to these putative fathers, washing clothes for the children is mostly done by the mothers. Only five of the seventeen fathers said they provided this service themselves. In the remaining cases, the fathers admitted that the service was provided by the grandparents of the child.

The children are washed about equally by mother and father. In some cases, they share this chore. As to who buys soap, twelve fathers reported that they bought it. This may because fathers have greater access to financial resources than mothers. On the other hand, it may be based on the reality that quite often, when fathers do contribute to the maintenance of children they are not living with, they frequently do so in the form of cash. This can be used to buy supplies such as soap and this is what the men assumed. Asked about who buys books, most fathers did not reply. It may be that the children were too young to go to school. Only four fathers said they bought books. The same number of fathers said they take care of school fees as well as school uniforms. It is interesting to note that putative fathers give greater credit to themselves than to the mothers. However, this is not surprising. Family studies in other parts of the world indicate that parents tend to overestimate their own contribution or differ in their perceptions of their relative contributions. This is not to say that anybody is necessarily lying.

Access and custody

In Kibaha, all teenage mothers lived with their children either alone, with the putative father, or with grandparents and other relatives. None of the putative fathers lived with the illegitimate child without its mother. In one case, a father had made a request to take his 10-year-old son into his custody. However, the son's mother, who had been a teenager when he was born, referred the man to her maternal uncles in Lindi where she hails from. She explained to me that according to her people's customs, such a father would have to plead his case and may have to pay compensation to the uncles for their maintenance expenses. The irony of the situation is that it was not the teenage mother who was to be compensated but her maternal uncles, although the son had been under the guardianship of the mother most of the time. The mother is now a trained nurse, has never married, and has another child out-of-wedlock.

Profile of care in Bunju

Eleven teenage mothers were interviewed randomly in Bunju ward near Bagamoyo district. One mother said she is assisted by her own mother with whom she lives in caring for her child. Another is assisted by her current husband while yet another is assisted by her father, with whom she lives. The remaining eight said they were taking care of their children alone. All except one who was married, lived with their parents.

Asked as to who takes care of their children while they (teenage mothers) worked away from home, four mentioned their own mothers. It was only the married teenage mother who said she was helped by her husband, even though he is not the father of the child. Another mentioned her grandmother while yet another mentioned her father and mother jointly. Two of the teenage mothers said they took care of their children while working outside the home.[19] Two other teenage mothers were casually employed in peasant agriculture (*vibarua*). Other activities mentioned included petty trade, peasant farming, and selling buns.

Fathers accepted paternity in all cases in Bunju. Six of the eleven women said that the putative fathers were not assisting in any way to maintain the children. In three cases, the putative fathers were assisting only occasionally. In two cases, the putative fathers had custody of the children and were, therefore, providing for them in most respects. This latter situation was particularly interesting considering that the inhabitants of Bunju, like those in neighbouring Bagamoyo, are supposedly matrilineal. Among the three who acknowledged the putative father's help in raising the children, two said the fathers were giving them money while another said the father helped when she was down on her luck.

Regarding the assistance of parents, five of the eleven mothers said their parents helped to obtain food, clothes, shelter, and medical facilities for their children. Medical facilities were frequently emphasized, indicating both that the children were often sick and that health care was considered to be costly in the area. Another said her parents gave her money to buy other necessities in addition to food and medical care. Three teenage mothers said they had not received any kind of assistance from their parents.

Prodded as to whether there were other relatives who helped them besides their own parents, six teenage girls said they were not receiving any assistance from other relatives. They either underwrote everything themselves or were helped by their own parents only. The other five teenage girls received assistance from other relatives such as a sister or aunt for clothes, washing, food, and medical facilities; a brother who provided for everything and particularly medical facilities; a sister who took the child to live with her; and an uncle who gave her money to buy maize flour for porridge when the mother had no money.

---

[19] Petty trade was the major income generating activity undertaken by six of the eleven teenage mothers in Bunju.

Access and custody

Bunju was slightly different from Kibaha. There is no social welfare office (SWO) in the area but the functions of the SWO are performed by community based officers (CBOs) attached to local government. In the absence of the SWO, teenage mothers, their relatives, and some of the putative fathers were identified through the CBOs. These officers are in effect voluntary extension workers living in the community. The story of one woman, a former teenage mother, highlighted some of the factors affecting teenage mothers' choices on custody and access to their children born out-of-wedlock. She has six children out-of-wedlock. Most of them do not have the same father.

> I decided to live with my children for better or for worse. ... One man by whom I had two children lives with them. He took them at the age 1 1/2 years. He lives with them here in Bunju. They are Zaramo. Their father and his people take them to school and provide them with everything. The children come to me if they have problems, such as the need for uniforms. They also come to visit. We are on good terms with their father. He tells me when there is a problem. For example, last December he was sick, so he asked me to buy uniforms for them because he was not working. I did. But now he is well and has taken over the responsibility to care for them. I have no obligation to do anything for these two children under this arrangement.

As to why she allowed only this father to take the children and not the others, her answer revealed economic considerations. The father of the children has a wholesale shop for foodstuffs. His father (grandparent) sells fish at Kariakoo market, the trading centre of Dar es Salaam.

> The grandfather used to live with the children's (paternal) grandmother, but some time ago he married another wife. This grandmother left with my children and lived with their father. They are taking good care of the children. I knew they had the means *(wana uwezo)*, that is why I allowed them to take my children.

Thus, a putative father's custody of, and access to children born out-of-wedlock may depend on many factors, including the financial ability of the putative father, the willingness of his relatives to help, and goodwill between the putative father and mother. In this particular case, the putative father had not yet married and he had no other children.

Tatu explains why she refused to give custody of her other son when he was a 6-year-old, to his father: "The father of my 14-year-old son wanted to take him at about the age of five or six years. I refused because he had disputed paternity from the beginning. Now he was coming forward because the child was old enough to run errands. I refused."

Asked what would happen if the father decided to fight for custody of his son even at that late hour, she said he could not claim this because he had not married her. This statement is generally true. In all cases in Kibaha, Bunju, and Kagera, fathers who got custody or parental access to their children born out-of-wedlock while their mothers were young and unmarried were either economically much better off than the mothers, or the mothers' parents conceded their inability to take care of the child and its teenage mother. When parents of the girl are very poor, or her home environment is unstable, the girl or her parents are generally desperate to have the putative father take custody of the child.

In one case in Bunju, a putative father described how he obtained custody. He is a watchman at the vegetable garden belonging to someone in Dar es Salaam. The boy's own home is Kibiti area in Rufiji district, also in the Coast region. He came to Bunju because he was hired by his boss through relatives in Rufiji.

> During my stay here I made a girl pregnant. Her parents were uncooperative, they sent her to me. But my financial position does not allow me to take care of the three of us. So I sent her to live with my mother in Rufiji. She now has an 8-month-old baby. They live in Rufiji while I live here.

When asked whether he had married her, he said he had not. "I have not married her because my present economic position does not allow me to marry. When the situation permits, I will marry another woman. I would have married her but her parents do not want me to."

The girl was not there to corroborate the details. However, I wondered whether she and her family did not consider her as being married. Living with the man's parents while the man migrates in search of wage employment, particularly where the two have a child together, is considered to be evidence of marriage in many parts of the country. Yet the man is right, for according to the law he is not married. His mother may know that but find it convenient to have the teenage mother around to assist her in her farming activities and, of course, take care of her infant child. It is unlikely that such a live-in mother would be allowed to leave the putative father's parents' home with her child after it is weaned. There are some opportunity costs involved. She may have earned a place to live and assistance in raising her child, but she has to live in a maid/helping hand relationship and possibly lose her right to custody. Moreover, if the putative father's fortunes do not improve, and there is no reason to assume that they will, he may end up marrying her because she is the stick in hand.[20]

As a matter of fact, it is arguable that their relationship may qualify for presumption of marriage under S. 160 of *LMA*, which provides that when a woman has lived with a man for at least two years and they have acquired the reputation of husband and wife in their community, they will be presumed to be married for the purposes of division of matrimonial assets on divorce or separation.

Finally, I asked participants at a focus group discussion about their views on maintenance of children born out-of-wedlock to teenage girls. Their responses were varied but all except one called for intervention by the government, religious institutions, donors, and individuals with higher incomes *(watu wenye uwezo)*, in that order, to help care for such children.

- The government, donors and religious institutions should devise means, such as loans, to help the mothers to generate incomes of their own;
- We should not rely on the putative fathers because they have proved to be negligent in caring for their children;
- Mothers of such children should settle down so that they can get men to marry them and they can lead happy lives for their children and themselves. The sole married teenage mother in Bunju pointed out that this would save the woman from contracting incurable medical diseases such as AIDS.

Kagera region

Kagera region is composed of five districts. Of these five districts, I visited Muleba and Bukoba. The latter is the headquarters for the region, including the regional SWO. Previously, the bulk of its cases had

---

[20] After a Swahili proverb: *Fimbo iliyo mbali haiui nyoka* ("The stick that is not near cannot help you kill a snake").

been affiliation-related and, as on the Coast, the office tended to serve the population of the urban and surrounding areas. Moreover, with the AIDS pandemic, the SWO in Kagera had undergone some reorganization. In order to deal with the influx of widows and orphans, a district SWO had been instituted in the two study areas. Unfortunately, the two offices were still caught up in the reorganization process and I was not able to benefit from the institutional data base.[21] I chose two wards in Muleba and Bukoba rural districts. These were Buganguzi in Muleba and Kishanje in Bukoba. As in the Coast region, comparability guided me. I anticipated that when the results were compared and contrasted they would provide a more telling picture of present trends among the Bahaya, the inhabitants of these areas.

Muleba district is home to many migrant settlers from Bukoba and the other neighbouring districts of Biharamulo and Ngara, and even countries like Rwanda and Burundi. Perhaps because of this intermingling with non-indigenous people, the area gives the impression of being less conservative about maternal custody and care of legitimate children. I considered it useful to find out the trends with respect to illegitimate children and whether this has any impact on the lives of teenage girls.

Care of children, custody, and access

Comparing the Coast region with Kagera, it was more difficult to identify putative fathers in the latter region. Within Kagera region itself, it was more difficult to identify putative fathers in Bukoba's rural areas than in Muleba district. There were cases of girls who have had children out-of-wedlock. Nonetheless, these were very few especially in Kishanje ward in Bukoba district as compared to Buganguzi ward in Muleba district and even more so to Kibaha and Bunju. Only one putative father was identified in Muleba, and information about him had to be taken for whatever it is worth. Moreover, this information was obtained indirectly, by interviewing his female relatives and brother-in-law. It was explained to me that making a young unmarried girl pregnant carries a stigma both for the men and the women concerned. It is considered shameful. Although sexual rela-

---

[21] Under pressure from AIDS-related NGOs and because of community crises, the office is now more focused on widows and orphans but affiliation of children is still one of its main functions under the Department of Family and Children.

tions cannot be said to be especially restrictive—some would say it is traditionally more permissive among the Bahaya than in many patrilineal societies—yet it is considered a "game for grown ups".

This one putative father, Kazoba, was 30 years old and was 25 when the child was born. He is Mhaya by ethnic origin, born in the ward, a peasant, and Christian. He was living with his child born out-of-wedlock and also with a woman by whom he had no child and to whom he was not married. The relatives said that the child was cared for by its father's live-in female partner while the father provided shelter and clothes. Food was obtained from subsistence farming. Clothes were washed by the stepmother, who also bathes the child. The father bought the soap.

The father never married. He was never charged in any institution to pay maintenance but the matter was amicably decided upon between the families; he himself, his parents and the girl's parents. His parents had never been to school and they were both peasants. They helped him with food, shelter, and clothes for the child when he and his child lived with them, but he moved out when his house was completed.

Profile of teenage mothers

Nine teenage mothers were interviewed. Their present ages ranged from 17 to 33 years. Only two were teenagers at the time of the study. Four women had been teenagers at the time of pregnancy. Looking at their level of education, most of the mothers were literate and had gone to the same school. Six had completed primary school, while one dropped out in Standard 6 and one had completed Form 4. The illiterate exception had never been to school. They were Christians, except one who said she had no religion. Seven were peasants, one a teacher, and another did not respond to this question.

Most of the mothers had only one child, while two other mothers had two children each. These children were born between 1980 and 1995. Five of the children stayed with their grandfathers: in effect, this may just mean that the children are living with their grandparents or that the grandmothers are divorced, separated, or widowed. As to who provides for the children, this was done by grandfathers for five children, grandmothers for two children, a mother for one and the putative father for another one. Clothing was provided by grandfathers in all cases.

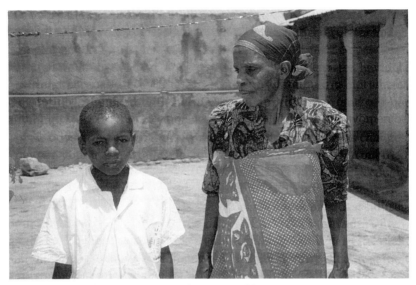

Many children are living with their grandparents or with (Photo Rita Liljeström)
their divorced, separated, or widowed grandmothers.

All but one mother obtained their food supplies from farming and the exception said she combined farming with buying. Bathing was done by the mothers in four cases, while washing clothes was done by grandmothers and mothers respectively. Six children had not started school but in the three cases where children had started schooling, school materials were provided by a grandfather or grandmother. The children's ages ranged from two months to 15 years and all of them were alive at the time of the study.

All the mothers were Bahaya born and bred in the neighbourhood. Of the nine, seven were not married while two were. Of the two married, one was in a monogamous relationship and she was the first wife, the other was in a polygamous marriage and she was the third wife.[22]

None of the seven unmarried mothers had plans for marriage. None of them was engaged in any income generating activity either. Regarding the putative fathers, they were not known in eight of the cases.[23] This answer was derived by asking villagers as to whether

---

[22] This is considered degrading for a girl among the Bahaya unless a man is very prosperous.

[23] This question was not put to mothers directly on advice from my contacts because of its sensitivity.

they knew the names of the fathers born to so and so. One mother said she knew the co-parent of her child and he was the one living with the child. They said there was no institutional forum in which to press claims for maintenance and in any case, even if there were, they thought the fathers would just refuse, thereby bringing more shame onto the women. Eight of the girls had at least one surviving parent. The fathers of eight of them had completed primary education, but the mothers of six had never been to school while one had reached Standard 4. Two did not answer this question because their mothers were dead. Regarding assistance received from relatives, mostly parents, it was in the form of food, clothing, lodging, medical care, and education.

Relatives' perspectives

Seven parents and relatives of the teenage mothers were interviewed. Their ages ranged from 54 to 70 years of age. All of them were peasants. They all had children who bore children as teenagers and they said that they assisted their grandchildren as best they could but they were all concerned about the future of their daughters. Their concern hinged on the diminishing chances of their daughters getting married. The parents said they would have helped their daughters to go after the putative fathers by taking their girls to those men, but lamented that the culprits were not known.

The stories of two former teenage mothers, Agatha and Theofilda, give a clearer indication of the situation in this area. They had subsequently married but had to leave their children born out-of-wedlock with their own parents. All the remaining seven of the nine teenage mothers interviewed were unmarried and lived with their children in the homes of their own parents or grandparents or great-grandparents. For those two who managed to get married, one was married to a polygamist and another to a single but much older man who had returned to the village after a long absence.

Bukoba: Kishanje

Kishanje ward in Bukoba rural district, on the lake border with Uganda, has been closed to migration. It was selected for its traditional, conservative outlook towards premarital fertility and the prevailing fear of losing land to newcomers in form of maternal offspring (*abaiwa*). In the Kishanje ward, of the five out-of-wedlock mothers identified by my contacts, only one was actually a teenage mother. She had married after the birth of her child but was later blamed for the calamity which befell her affinal family when three of her subsequent children died. She was expelled from both her natal and marital home, and ordered to pay a "fine" to cleanse the family and stop the misfortune. She needed to buy a goat for this ritual, but in the process of raising the money, she met a migrant labourer from Burundi who now cohabits with her and her illicit child. The migrant labourer may not share the cultural beliefs of the local inhabitants and such people are considered to be of lower social and economic status. The child is now 6 years old, an age at which he can assist with errands for his mother and stepfather. The mother was 17 when he was born. She is an orphan.

Sources of maintenance for infants: An overview

In the few cases where putative fathers contributed to the maintenance of their children born out-of-wedlock, the contribution was often in the form of cash. The sources of cash for some of the putative fathers interviewed included farming but also petty trade, quarrying, casual labour, and wages in Bunju. Others were formally employed as traders, welders, and peasant farmers. Putative fathers were evasive in Kishanje ward, but based on information derived from teenage mothers, they were farmers, students, traders, and wage earners. In Muleba, only one putative father was identified and he was a farmer.

The sources of cash for those teenage mothers who said they had any included the sale of agricultural produce and cooked food, and wages in Kibaha and Bunju. There were also those engaged in bartending, saloon work, and hospital employment in Kibaha. In Muleba and Bukoba, most mothers were peasants, with the exception of two primary school teachers. The case studies revealed both the specificity of individual teenage mothers and the generality of their predicament.

Among the five families selected in Kibaha, one family was caring for three infant children born to its two teenage daughters. The girls just sat there with their other siblings and parents and fed their infants whatever food the girls' father managed to bring. Their mother also admitted to not being engaged in any kind of activity that would generate food for the family. The man was a retired watchman and had managed to secure a place and build a seven-room mud and thatched roof house in an L shape. They had ten children of their own, none of whom was gainfully employed. The eldest son had an auxiliary job, but had recently been retrenched. Moreover, the family was so poor and food deficient that they were obliging the older children to take responsibility for some of the younger ones, although the former were unemployed. It was interesting that this family so un-grudgingly looked after its illegitimate children. However, the parents had contributed to their daughter's situation. They had encouraged their daughters to cohabit with their boyfriends in the family com-pound in the hope that they would marry their daughters. Both these men had formally been in the army at a nearby barracks, and they brought home some foodstuffs such as meat, rice, and sugar in the beginning. However, these men left after the girls became pregnant. One had lived with the girl at the barracks, but brought her back claiming that his wife had returned from his home village. Prodded as to why they had not insisted on a formal marriage before being taken for a ride, as they obviously were, they said they had been fooled by the prospective suitors' payment of a customary engagement sum of 200 shillings, which is as good as marriage along the coast. However, the men were from Songea in the southern part of the country, which is patrilineal and does not have this custom.

The second family in Kibaha comprised a single mother of two children who had her first child out-of-wedlock when she was a teen-ager. She is in her early 30s. She is formally employed as a nurse/midwife and her first child is now a teenager. He is the son whose father was reported to have been referred to his mother's maternal uncles in Lindi. So far, the putative father has been paying mainten-ance in kind rather than cash. Such payments included a tin of maize, or a bag of maize flour. Although the mother rents two rooms in a mud house, there was no doubt that she was living below standard for her job. The father was married to another woman. Her eldest son was on probation with the social welfare office for truancy. At the time of my research, she had a 3-year-old toddler, whom she said she had after giving up hope of marriage.

The third family comprised a successful single mother of six, who also had her first child when she was a teenager. She is managing her family with the help of a thriving agricultural produce sales business near the Morogoro Road, which she runs partly on a cooperative basis with other women (*upatu*). In her case, the difference was that her father gave her land of her own after the birth of her first child. She launched a prolonged affiliation claim after which she was awarded what she considered an unsatisfactory amount. She has long stopped to bothering about the meagre social welfare instalments paid by the father of one of her sons because it was cumbersome to follow up.

The fourth family consisted of a teenage mother who had two children by two different men, who were formally employed by the neighbourhood bank and prison respectively. Both parents of the teenage mother were formally employed. The father had filed a claim in the social welfare office against the two men for compensation for what he called the pollution (*uchafuzi*) of his daughter. He claimed compensation for himself and not maintenance for his grandchildren. This went beyond the mandate of the social welfare office presiding over the case, which is to assist in collecting maintenance for children in problematic situations such as this one. Moreover, according to the social welfare officials, the meeting broke down because the father and daughter began a heated argument and switched to the vernacular. They had not returned to the office by the end of my research.

In the fifth family, the teenage mother and putative father cohabited yet the woman continued to collect maintenance instalments from the social welfare office. The woman is fully aware that she is not married and considers this advantageous to her child. She said, "Being married, even living with the man, is no guarantee he will spend money on the child. He can drink it or give it to other women. But when I get money from the social welfare office I buy what the child needs."

In her view, this is the advantage of not being legally married. She assumes the social welfare office does not know that the two parents live together, and hence enforces the maintenance agreement. In fact, the office does know, and the officers are pleased with the arrangement particularly because the man is paying his instalments faithfully.

Institutional support for the mother and her kin

As stated earlier, the official institutional support provided by the law in affiliation cases is the social welfare office. Moreover, traditionally in many communities, it is the youth's family, particularly the girl's, regulated by the clan or extended family, who deal with such close personal matters. Where the community is made up of migrants from different parts of the country, as it is in Kibaha, the social welfare office steps into the shoes of the clan on behalf of the state.

In the studied regions, the social welfare offices were well established in regional headquarters. Consequently, the areas near the regional headquarters were better served than more distant areas. The reason for this distribution of services may be pragmatic, to minimize costs. Moreover, it is normally the urban area near regional headquarters which is likely to have a population with loose family ties and hence be in greater need of a social support system. The latter is demonstrated by the enormous number of affiliation cases in Kibaha, which was not the case in other areas.

Between the years 1990–93, there were thirty-seven affiliation cases in Kibaha, both for teenage and adult women. We have seen how some of these women were assisted by the social welfare office to obtain the contributions of putative fathers to the maintenance of their infant children. That is not to say that there were no enforcement problems. Indeed, several problems and complaints were levelled against these offices. Some of the complaints from the community as highlighted in focus group discussions were, lack of authority to enforce compliance, favouritism towards putative fathers, and corruption. But one officer articulated the dilemma of the social welfare office thus:

> Having children out-of-wedlock is deviant behaviour for both men and women. The social welfare office's role is to listen to both parties and try to help them reach an amicable settlement. But women often break down during the proceedings. When they speak they start crying. The men gain extra confidence and charge, "You are the one who has called me. Speak (*sema sasa*). I have no ability to pay maintenance (*Sina uwezo*)." The women expect us to sympathize and favour them. But that is not our role.

The role of the social welfare office was explained as one of conciliation rather than applying the law. Unlike the courts, whose role is to apply the law to the facts of the case, the SWO applies community values whereby people are to be made to feel equal to each other and are encouraged to be mutually concerned about their problems. The officers contended that this approach is best where children are concerned because it creates an environment in which parents can actually cooperate in the upbringing of their child. They also defended themselves against allegations that they accuse parents of complacency and greed by pointing out that sometimes it is necessary to waken parents to reality. They gave examples of misuse of maintenance instalments by girls' parents, such as "we have lived with the child all this time. It ate our food, why should maintenance money be spent solely on the child?" Instead, the child's money becomes the family's money.

The SWO has no powers to force parties to comply, so that if parties cannot agree, they are referred to court and the office is often called to give evidence in such cases. One could say that the SWO is intended to take over the crumbling role of the elders under traditional custom by looking after the welfare of the entire community in the country as one big family.

The family is the first institution. We learn basic values from the family and tend to treasure most of these values for life. The family is also expected to protect its members, especially children, when these values are threatened. Moreover, customs have changed in modern times. Elders and religious leaders no longer have the moral leadership they had even as late as in the 1950s and 1960s. Parents are not necessarily desirable role models for their children. Poverty has demoralized many parents. They cannot provide adequately for their families and, therefore, cannot honestly deny some of the desires of their children. They see these as aspirations to upward social mobility. For example, in a poor urbanized family where no adult is gainfully employed, the parents understand that when their daughters run after salaried or otherwise successful males with money, they are trying to escape the poverty in which they were raised. Somehow deep inside, parents hope with their children that they will succeed. This theme was echoed in different guises in all the research areas.

Subsequent marriage of the mother

Most of the women had not married after giving birth to children out-of-wedlock. This may be indicative of the difficulty a girl who has a child out-of-wedlock later has in getting married. They probably give up hope as their age advances or are scared of the responsibility and trouble after their first experience of raising a child. It is also possible that prospective suitors did not materialize. As one former teenage mother who is a nurse commented in Kibaha, she waited ten years after her first child to get married. She later gave up and decided to have another child.

The issue of men's seeming lack of interest in committing themselves to marriage came up again and again in the focus group discussions. In Kibaha, some of the explanations were the high cost of bridewealth, the cost of the wedding, and tribalism. In the latter case, it is a situation of the girl's or boy's parents insisting that one should marry within the ethnic group. Sometimes, parents want their grown child to marry a particular child to create a lasting relationship with a well placed family. When youths are in love, they may end up having a child, but they lack the courage to disobey their parents, or they may even fall out with their partners, before making firm commitments to them.

In Bunju, the boys' reluctance to marry was bitterly complained of by the mothers of the girls. They said the boys were behaving irresponsibly by making the girls pregnant and avoiding shouldering the burden of parenting by claiming they had no income. They wondered why they continued to chase the girls. They also blamed the girls for being vain and wanting what they should not have.

On the other hand, the boys and the adult men charged that the girls preferred highly mobile boyfriends, drivers of cars or motorbikes from Dar es Salaam, rather than local boys. As a result, local men felt marginalized and blamed this on unemployment and the resultant economic deprivation.

The girls blamed everybody, the men for being dishonest and deceitful, and the mothers for not understanding that things have changed. They gave several examples, such as men promising to marry the girl after the child was born but abandoning her in the seventh month of pregnancy. Another was refusing to contribute regularly to maintenance. Last but not least was the allegation that the boys habitually burst condoms during sexual intercourse. One girl claimed to have fallen pregnant when the man she slept with was supposed to be wearing a condom. After a heated discussion with the entire workshop forum, she stood up and said, "Look, we love you *(tunawapenda)*, our local boys, but you cannot maintain us. We could all be having fun and not sitting here blaming each other, but you have to be considerate of our needs *(mahitaji yetu)."*

For their part, the adult men blamed the government for its recent cost-sharing policy which resulted in cuts to social service expenditures especially health and education. They said this has demoralized the men and was responsible for their reluctance to marry. One man alleged, "When you touch a woman *(ukimgusa tu mwanamke)*, the next day she is at your doorstep asking for money to go to hospital. Then she needs to go to the clinic. Before you know it she has a child and endless medical bills and requests for more money."

Summary

This chapter and the study on which it is based is an attempt to shed light on the role of the law in the care of children born out-of-wedlock to teenage mothers. We have seen that although the law does not define care, the communities bringing up these children understand what it means and do what they can to bring children up. Teenage mothers and generally their own relatives have custody of and access to the children, not because of any legal benefit but because nobody else wants or contests the custody of the children. There were a few cases where fathers had custody of the children in special circumstances. However, as mothers and their relatives crave to share this responsibility with the putative fathers, fathers did not complain of custody or access being denied them.

The sources of monetary settlement for infants' needs were varied but depended on who was providing the settlement and the area in which they lived. In Kagera, the fathers provided support mostly from wages, while mothers obtained it mainly by trade in the informal sector. Other sources included grandparents of the children. In Kagera, the source of monetary settlements was mostly farming.

The institutional support received by the mothers included the family and the social welfare office. The latter was much more effective, as illustrated by the case studies in Kibaha where the office was fully functional. It was in this area that the law was at least felt in the community, while in the other research areas the community was having to make do outside the legal regime. Moreover, the family, while often helping with basic logistical support, was not successful in helping mothers to obtain maintenance for children from putative fathers. It is also noteworthy that the extended family was more effective in Kagera, even at the level of grand- and great-grandparents, whereas along the coast only the immediate family played a role. Nonetheless, one notes that aunts and sisters did not feature in Kagera, probably because women are less autonomous in patrilineal rural communities than in urban and peri-urban areas, with their more socially relaxed matrilineal moves.

Finally, it was noted that the chances of subsequent marriage by former teenage mothers are low. For those few who have married, they have had to leave their children with their parents and grandparents in Kagera, although another was able to take her child into a marriage in Bunju.

It is therefore, clear that the law is remote from the actual problems of the community, not because it is irrelevant, but because of the lack of an effective administrative network that spans the entire countryside. There is no doubt that such machinery is essential, as evidenced by the fear of even mentioning putative fathers in Kagera. Without such administrative machinery, it is unlikely that meaningful discourse on sharing responsibility for children born out-of-wedlock will even begin, and teenage mothers will continue to bear the full load.

References

Dahl, S.T., 1987, *Women's Law. An Introduction to Feminist Jurisprudence*. Oslo: Norwegian University Press.

Freeman, M., 1984, "Questioning the de-legalization movement in Family Law. Do we really want a family court?", in Eekelar, J. and S. Katz (eds.), *The Resolution of Family Conflicts*.

James R.W. and G.M. Fimbo, 1973, *Customary Law of Tanzania: A Source Book*. Nairobi: East African Literature Bureau.

Maidement, S., 1984, *Child Custody and Divorce: The Law in Social Context*. London: Croom Helm.

Mongulla, B., 1991, "Children under Especially Difficult Circumstances in Tanzania: The Case of Street Children". Unpublished report for UNICEF Tanzania.

Mwakanjala, T.E., 1993, "Problems and Dilemma of Street Children in Tanzania. A Case Study of Dar es Salaam Region". Unpublished M.A. thesis, Department of Development Studies, University of Dar es Salaam.

Rwebangira, M.K., 1988, "Women's Priorities for Legal Reform in Tanzania". Paper presented to the UNICEF Tanzania office's Task Force on Women in November 1988.

Rwebangira, M.K., 1991, "Women's Priorities for Legal Reform in Tanzania". Paper written for UNICEF Task Force on Women and published by TAMWA in *Sauti ya Siti*, January–March 1991, Dar es Salaam.

—1992a, "Legal Aspects of Teenage Girls' Reproductive Health in Tanzania: A Look at Contraception, Abortion and Infanticide". Teenage Girls' Reproductive Health Study Group, Women's Research and Documentation Project, University of Dar es Salaam.

—1992b, "Women Seeking Redress in Court of Law in Tanzania: A Survey of Mbeya and Dar es Salaam Regions". Unpublished Research Report for the Organization of Social Science Research in Eastern Africa.

—1995, "Legal Status of Women and Poverty". Paper presented at the Socio-Economic Growth and Poverty Alleviation in Tanzania Workshop jointly organized by the Government of Tanzania and the World Bank, Arusha, 14–20 May, 1995.

—1996, *Legal Status of Women and Poverty in Tanzania.* Research Report No. 100. Uppsala: The Nordic Africa Institute.

Rwezaura, B.A., 1985, *Traditional Family Law and Change in Tanzania. A study of Kuria Social System.* Hamburg University.

—1986–7, "More Protection of Children in Tanzania", *Journal of Family Law,* Vol. 25:261–67.

— and U. Wanitzek, 1988, "The Law and Practice Relating to the Adoption of Children", *Tanzania Journal of African Law,* 32, 2.

Smart, C., 1989, *Feminism and the Power of Law.* London and New York: Routledge.

—and S. Sevenhuijsen, 1989, *Child Custody and the Politics of Gender.* London and New York: Routledge.

Swantz, M.L., 1985, *Women in Development: A Creative Role Denied? The Case of Tanzania.* London: C. Hurst & Company and New York: St. Martin's Press.

ANNEX TO CHAPTER 7

RECOMMENDATIONS

Sensitizating communities to the needs of the current reality

Sensitization of communities at village and ward levels to deal with the current reality of children born out-of-wedlock rather than romanticizing the past or condemning the present. This would need intervention programmes to help communities focus on their strengths and assess their weaknesses with a view to devising practicable local solutions within broad national policies and laws, without undue reliance on the central government and courts. This can be done through the Village Government and Community Development Officers whose network extend to village level.

2. Strengthening village governments

Village governments are closer to the people and can be strengthened to support teenage mothers and their families by getting putative fathers to share in the responsibilities of raising children born out-of-wedlock. This would involve both formal and informal aspects of intervention, unlike the present situation where teenage mothers who live in remote areas not served by the Social Welfare Office are left to suffer alone with their parents.

3. Enlarging the scope of children's rights

In many Tanzanian societies there are many good and positive norms expressed in proverbs and folk stories that cherish children. Communities could be encouraged to capture these sentiments which complement national law and the Convention on the Rights of the Child. Such a move could also help to improve national laws on children, which remain fragmented and largely unfocused at present.

4. Adequate and accessible legal services at national level

If maintenance claims are to be taken seriously, credible collection and enforcement mechanisms must to be put in place in all areas of the country. At the national level, the legal profile of dealing with maintenance of children born out-of-wedlock or on the break up of marriage should be raised by amending the Affiliation Ordinance to deal with current socio-economic conditions, including the human rights of women and children.

5. Family life education should include family responsibility

In those schools where family life education (FLE) is finally being offered, the curriculum should go beyond sex education and prevention of STDs to include mutual respect and at least the intention of making long term commitments to the partner and to the child which may be born as a result of intercourse. Emphasis should be placed on the values of abstinence and postponement of sexual intercourse until such time "as the parties are" ready and able to take responsibility for their actions. This is the message contained in the curriculum of traditional initiation ceremonies of many of the country's societies. The idea is to spread the positive message to the rest of the country.

Chapter 8
Stone-Breakers and Brick-Lifters Aspiring for Earnings and Families

Mary Ntukula

In the rural areas agricultural labour is seasonal, and not all seasons are conducive to crop growing. Consequently, teenage girls flock to towns to look for the possibilities of work in the formal sector or in service, or for doing menial work. However, these sectors cannot absorb all of them. Therefore, young women resort to looking for available work in other fields like construction, as stone-breakers and even as coolies. They opt for such employment so they can survive and support their families—parents and siblings—and most importantly, to become economically empowered, "empowerment" being the slogan of the day. These rural teenage girls have a low economic status, little education, and they have had less access to technical schooling than young men. This makes their job prospects very limited. Like any human beings, the young women want to be able to marry and have children, to make ends meet, and to lead their own lives. The present chapter gives an account of the aspirations of and harsh realities facing thirty teenage girls who migrated from the rural regions to the city. It is based on interviews and observations at quarries and construction sites

Songea, Ruvuma region, and Dar es Salaam

Songea is the regional headquarters of Ruvuma region, which is in southern Tanzania. The main economic activity of Ruvuma region is agriculture. Major cash crops are tobacco, maize, and coffee. Food crops include beans and maize. Ruvuma is one of four major grain producing areas in Tanzania. During the colonial period, Ruvuma region was isolated. It had a poor infrastructure compared to other regions. Consequently, Songea grew very slowly. According to the 1982 Mlale resolution, not much construction was undertaken at the time.

After independence, the situation improved. The all-weather trunk road was built from Dar es Salaam during the early 1980s. Likewise, the Uhuru railway, which had been completed by the 1970s, made communication with the region easier. Songea, which was once neglected, started to grow faster and faster. Schools, houses, shops, and hotels were now being built at an ever increasing rate. The Mlale resolution resolved that every indigenous Ruvuma inhabitant should build him or herself a permanent house. Also a strategy was devised to improve roads within the region and those linking the region with other regions. As a result, local people started to build their own houses using permanent building materials like bricks, cement, and corrugated iron sheets. This trend was coupled with an influx of women into the construction industry. These women were aged between 15 and 55 years. Their occupations on these construction sites range from physical labour like lifting bricks, making concrete, and fetching water to selling foodstuffs to labourers.

Dar es Salaam is the capital of Tanzania. It serves as both the centre of political administration in the country and as its a commercial centre. The city is growing fast, with many new buildings mushrooming. There are also many other construction works, including roads and houses, especially in the suburbs. This means that there is a high demand for quarried stone and aggregates.

The main quarry areas in Dar es Salaam are Kigamboni, Msasani, Masaki, Kunduchi, and Oysterbay. These areas are on the shores of the Indian Ocean and they are rich in coral reefs. They are also inhabited, and people live everywhere around them. When these residents garden, they dig out the coral rocks and throw them away. Men come and collect the rocks, fill their carts with them, and sell the stones and rocks to the women, including teenage girls, who crush them into smaller stones. They afterwards sell them to customers who use them for construction. Some of the rocks are directly obtained by digging in these areas.

I also observed during my fieldwork that when the Ali Hassani Mwinyi road was undergoing repairs, the men hastened to collect stones, probably to sell them to the women at the Namanga site, which the road passes. At that time the cost for one cart of stones was 1,000 shillings up to 2,000 shillings (about 3 and 6 US dollars).

These developments in Songea and Dar es Salaam prompted me to study on relationship between marriage, childbearing, and the rearing roles of teenage girls and their work as stone-breakers and brick-lifters. I also wanted to find out whether the teenage manual workers believe they can form their own families. What are the constraints they face in the course of fulfilling the above roles?

Looking for employment

I approached teenage girls who worked in the construction and quarry sites in Songea and Dar es Salaam respectively, but who were not members of those communities. They were all outsiders who had come a long way to find job opportunities. Employment on construction sites was one opportunity available to newcomers in the city. Local urban people have their own way of meeting their needs and they do not have to work on those sites. The Dar es Salaam stone-breakers had followed when their parents or husbands-to-be had moved to the city to escape rural unemployment. Only a few girls came on their own. Zaina, a 17-year-old girl, explained with tears rolling down her cheeks that she had followed her husband from Morogoro city. Her husband worked with the Ministry of Home Affairs, but unluckily he died after only one year of marriage. Zaina had to resort to stone-breaking in order to make a living. Ndikwija, another girl, chose to stay in Dar es Salaam and engage in stone-breaking work, in spite of her parents' decision to go back to their home village in Morogoro.

Table 1 shows the region of origin of the teenage girls and the distance from Dar es Salaam.

Table 1. *Region and distance from Dar es Salaam*

Place	Estimated distance from Dar es Salaam	Number of girls
Morogoro	200 km	3
Tanga	400 km	3
Pwani	100 km	1
Iringa	505 km	2
Kigoma	1,647 km	1
Dodoma	497 km	2
Mbeya	885 km	1
Mtwara	368 km	2
Total		15

On the other hand, most brick-lifters in Songea had migrated from rural villages within the region, either following their husbands or husbands-to-be, or their parents.

Table 2. *Region and distance from Songea*

Place	Estimated distance from Songea	Number of girls
Namtumbo	75 km	2
Peramiho	12 km	3
Liuli	120 km	2
Mgazani	15 km	1
Litoa	15 km	2
Mbinga Mharule	30 km	1
Matetereka	80 km	1
Gumbiro	90 km	1
Hanga	50 km	1
Madaba	150 km	1
Total		15

When the teenagers arrive in the city, everybody thinks of them as *washamba*, i.e., non-urbanites, people who are not familiar with the urban way of life or the tricks of the place. Upon arrival, some girls tried service jobs but ended up in stone-breaking and construction work after getting into trouble with their employers, often because of irregular pay. At this stage the girls feel uncertain as they do not have much support and security in the urban areas. After engaging in manual jobs, they regain confidence and begin to form their own support and security systems. They start by investigating their neighbourhood. Knowing their neighbours and interacting with them is crucial. Neighbours are expected to assist each other through difficult times before close relatives in the city or from the rural villages are contacted. Notwithstanding this, the teenage workers maintain ties with their places of origin as they expect to go back to the village if things do not work out in town or when they themselves get old.

How good are the girls' prospects for succeeding in town? What are their assets?

Education and prospects for employment

The educational level of most of the stone-breakers and brick-lifters ranged from zero to seven years of schooling. No one went to post-primary school. In most cases, they had completed Standard 7 at the age ranging from 14 to 16 years. A comparison reveals the following differences between girls in Songea and Dar es Salaam.

Table 3. *Teenage girl manual workers and their education levels*

Area	No education	Koranic	Std 1–4	Std 5–7	Total
Dar es Salaam	5	1	7	2	15
Songea	1	0	6	8	15
Total	6	1	13	10	30

More teenage workers from Songea have been educated to at least Standard 4 and 7, while the girls in Dar es Salaam had spent fewer years in primary school. A third of them had no formal education, and nearly half of the girls were educated only up to Standard 4. The differences can be attributed to the fact that most of the Dar es Salaam teenage girls have moved from up-country to look for menial jobs in the city after they realized that there is no future for them in the villages. Because of their low educational status they have to look for manual work. Although more Songea girls have a Standard 7 education, that level is still low and does not guarantee them employment in the formal sector.

While education is regarded as a good determinant of marriage age, in the case of these teenage girls, this connection was not clearly demonstrated. Although the girls completed school early, marriage is not their priority, especially not when they are preoccupied with their jobs in quarries and on the construction sites.

The brick-lifters in both Dar es Salaam and Songea saw education as a gender issue. Most of the girls said that they opted to do manual work because they lacked the education to secure jobs in the formal sector. When they were asked why they had a low education, most argued that their parents could not afford to educate them. Priority for receipt of meagre resources was given to the male children. An example of this is Mwajuma, a slim and tall teenage stone-breaker. At the time of the interview she was 19 years. Unfortunately, she could not go to school because her father had three wives and a limited income. His priority was to educate only the boys.

The lack of education was bitterly felt after the death of Mwajuma's father. Her life became unbearable. She decided to come to Dar es Salaam to look for employment as a house servant. She wanted to assist her mother, especially after the three huts which were left by her father had collapsed. At the time she was 15, she did housework for just a year, then met a man with whom she cohabited for two years. They had two children. Mwajuma hoped she would formalize her marriage to him, but the man left her when her second child was young. The man fell sick for a long time and died in 1993 after they had separated. She had to join the stone-breakers to earn money. When I asked her about her plans, she said she would not marry soon, although in future she might if she finds an appropriate partner. Mwajuma considers an appropriate partner to be one who can assist her during difficult times, such as when she is sick At the time I met her, she just had an operation and was still weak. Nevertheless, she had to continue to work in order to survive.

The working environment

In Dar es Salaam, we visited Oysterbay, Masaki, and Namanga quarries during our fieldwork. In total there were eighty-five women working in these quarries. Their ages ranged from 16 to 55. Only those who were under 20 were interviewed. The women use their hammers to make aggregates. They buy the big stones and rocks from their male suppliers, who carry the stones on their carts.

Most of the interviews were conducted at Namanga. The worksite of Namanga is located near the place where most of these teenage manual workers reside. According to a girl I interviewed, all her neighbours are stone-breakers. Teenage girls, their parents, or their husbands rent rooms in cheap makeshift houses. The houses are built of various materials ranging from mud to cement blocks. The roofs are mostly made of secondhand corrugated iron sheets. The walls in most cases are not plastered. The proximity of these houses is what matters to most of them because they can easily attend to their domestic chores as well as doing their jobs.

The place where the stone-breakers live at Namanga is bare, with hardly any trees and no shade. Scattered grass grows around the area, which is very dusty. The girls work with hammers from sunrise to sunset (6:00 a.m. to 6:00 p.m.) everyday, they break rocks on rainy and dry days, during hot and cold seasons. As a tall slender tall girl lamented, "We work everyday from morning till evening, come sun, come rain. We don't have Sundays or public holidays."

Sun and rain throughout the day without adequate clothing is not conducive to good health. Some young women do not understand the importance of wearing gloves to protect their hands or of using masks to prevent them from inhaling the dust produced by the stones. Even those who know the importance of protective gear, cannot afford to buy it. The teenage mothers bring their young children, who are exposed to the health hazards caused by the bad work environment and the poor working conditions. In visiting the areas, I always found children with runny noses, and I saw their mothers hastening to anyone stopping on the road, whether they are customers or not, shouting *Mteja, Malisafi* (an address to customers and quality goods, respectively).

In Songea, I started by identifying sites in which women worked. I was informed by the Songea UWT (*Umoja wa Wanawake wa Tanzania,* Union of Women of Tanzania) secretary that female manual workers in Songea work in quarries, on construction sites, and in tobacco godowns. There were six construction sites with a labour force which included both men and women from 15 to 55 years of age. UWT is a woman's organization affiliated to the main political party on Tanzania. According to the UWT chairperson of Songea branch, the men crush rocks with explosives. The women thereafter break the crushed rocks into smaller aggregates using hammers. This shows that the men have more access to technology than women. I managed to find four sites of the six which had a total of fifteen teenage girls, their ages ranging from 15 to 19 years. They were all interviewed.

On these construction sites, there was a clear division of labour between men and women. While men specialized in more technical jobs, such as laying the bricks and mixing concrete, the women, including the girls, simply carried the bricks, concrete, and water to the worksites. This could be attributed to the fact that men have a better chance of being trained in masonry than women, who seem to have entered this job market more recently than men. This situation was demonstrated by one of the teenage brick-lifters who commented, "If I had better technical training and education I would not be here carrying bricks on my head. Perhaps I would be laying bricks or even supervizing like the men are doing." This girl was quite determined to achieve more for herself.

It is also true that people generally do pay much regard to these women, as if nobody notices their existence in construction work. This fact was established during one of our workshops in Zanzibar. It

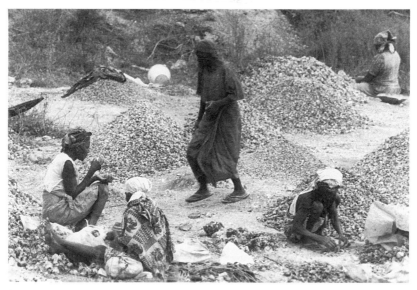

Stone-breakers in Dar es Salaam   (Photo Benny Kisanga)

appeared that workshop participants were not aware and could not
believe that women worked on construction sites. They had never
noticed them. To their surprize, when we walked out that same day
we, noticed some female workers on a site near our workshop venue.
They were busy mixing concrete, or carrying mixed concrete on their
heads, while others carried stones and bricks.

The working environment for the Songea girls is very harsh. Here
too they have to stay in the sun throughout the day, since the construction sites have no shade. There is no reliable and safe water. For
example at Mama Nashawa's plot in Songea I found girls drinking the
same water as was used for construction. They do not use protective
clothes, like caps and masks, to prevent them from inhaling cement
and dust. Neither do they have gloves. Some of them may not be
aware of the importance of the protective clothes. Even if they are
aware most of them have many other urgent needs. These teenage
workers do not have any security against sickness, pregnancy, or
when rearing young children. Given these difficult conditions and the
poor environment, it is to be expected that workers are prone to diseases, possibly occupational. Since teenagers are young and their
bodies are still growing, the work conditions could be particularly
hazardous to them.

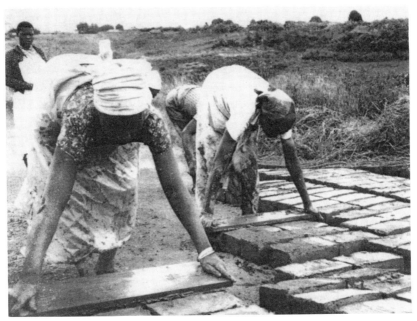

Women making bricks (*Pressphoto*, Dar es Salaam)

Ownership, organization of labour, and control of produce

The Dar es Salaam teenage stone-breakers have no source of income other than the money they earn from the aggregates. They but their stones. They themselves organize their work and they are the ones who appropriate the money from their labour. The women, including the teenage girls, have formed their own *ushirika* (cooperative association). If a member is sick or otherwise stuck, they all contribute to support her. This is an arrangement which provides security for members of the cooperative association (*wana ushirika*) during difficult times. The *wana ushirika* will sell the aggregates of a member who is sick or has some other problem and keep the money for her. *Ushirika* is not normally registered. When an *ushirika* is run by men, it is registered, and hence is protected by the law. Most women do not take the trouble to register their *ushirika*, hence the *ushirika* can change at any time or be manipulated in the interest of some members. The husbands of these girls have no share in this cooperative, through some of these teenagers obtain their capital from their husbands, parents, or relatives. Some obtain their capital from their former employers in the service sector.

In this manner, the teenage girls of Dar es Salaam have a say in and control over their produce. This was expressed by a short, fat, and strong girl thus: "After all this hard labour no one can dictate to me on how to use my money."

In my opinion, the teenage girls are economically empowered by being able to produce aggregate and earn their own income. The stone-breakers get a reasonably good income from their work: One of them gave me 400 shillings to buy a soft drink and pay for my busfare back home. When she opened her purse, I could see about 30,000 to 40,000 shillings inside. Both Dar es Salaam and Songea girls are cheerful and proud of their work. A Songea girl even turned down an offer of employment as a house servant, saying, "With this job I feel much more secure and I earn a more constant income than if I was employed as a house servant."

The stone-breakers do not think about taking on any other work. One of the Dar es Salaam girls commented:

> It is so convenient. I come here with my children. I have no obligations of hiring a babysitter. I can go home to prepare my food and do other household chores because my house is just a few metres away. In addition, my aggregate is in big demand. I am assured of some money everyday. It is not like selling buns—if you don't get customers, you have to throw them away, because they go stale. But with this business, the remaining aggregate can be sold a couple of days later without fear that it will rot.

The stone-breakers are the ones who determine the price of their aggregate. In this way they are not exploited.

I came across Hamisa, a smart 16-year-old girl with dark curly hair. She wore neat dresses and a piece of *khanga* around her waist while she worked. After work she would go for a walk and wear fashionable dresses. Hamisa was selling aggregate on part-time basis. During the morning, she did her nursing practice at a certain Bakwara (a Muslim organization) dispensary. During the evenings, she sold her aggregate. She told me that she was hoping to be employed as a nursing assistant in the autumn. She was very determined and seemed to like the job very much. She insisted that even if she secured the nursing job, she would continue to sell aggregate part-time. For her, it is good business. Hamisa earns about 2,000 shillings per day. She obtained her investment capital from her mother who worked on the same site. Hamisa left school in Standard 7.

Contrariwise, the Songea brick-lifters just own their labour power. They have to sell their labour on construction sites. In this way, they are much exploited. The owners of the buildings under construction are the ones who determine the rate of pay. They are paid 350 shillings per day, which is equivalent to 7,500 shillings per month (close to 50 US dollars at the time of my study). Their labour contract does not provide any security. When they are sick, they have to depend on their relatives. When they have an accident at work, their employers do not take any responsibility.

Male friends and prospects of marriage

Teenage stone-breakers in Dar es Salaam and brick-lifters in Songea alike not infrequently prefer to postpone marriage so they can earn at least some money and buy some essential items. Marriage, according to the teenage girls interviewed, is a situation in which male and female partners cohabit for more than a year and have an intimate relationship, or refers to those who are officially committed either through religious rites, Christian or Islamic, or through the area commissioner's office.

Table 4. *Age and marital status of teenage manual workers*

Study area	Age	Married	Single	Divorced	Widow	Total
Songea	15	-	1	-	-	1
	16	-	3	-	-	3
	17	1	1	-	-	2
	18	1	1	-	-	2
	19	2	3	2	-	7
Dar es Salaam	15	-	-	-	-	0
	16	-	-	-	-	0
	17	1	-	-	-	1
	18	4	2	1	1	8
	19	4	2	-	-	6
Total		13	13	3	1	30

Most of the teenage stone-breakers of Dar es Salaam were married (nine out of fifteen) while their counterparts, Songea brick-lifters, often stayed single (only four of fifteen were married). Of the 13 girls

who were married in Songea and Dar es Salaam, only four were officially married by either Christian or Islamic rites or in the area commissioner's office. The rest were cohabiting.

During the interviews, I found out that among the items that
teenage girls longed to posses in their lifetime were beds, sofas,
kitchen utensils, and in the long term, property like a house plot, a
small house, or a farm plot. Some girls were ambitious in that they
hoped to start some small project such as *mama ntilie,* i.e., preparing
and selling food on the streets. They wanted escape the burden of
their present jobs. Some of them wanted to marry after they achieved
their objectives. Others wished to marry in two or three years. As one
teenage girl argued: "I would like to postpone my marriage and
childbearing by two years, so that I can acquire assets. Who knows?
After marriage I might not have a say in my earnings." Those teenage
girls who express a wish to marry mostly think of marrying in three
years time. Since the majority of the unmarried girls were 17 to 19
years old at the time, this means they would marry at the age of 20 to
22 years.

In this way the girls find themselves in an ambiguous situation.
On the one hand, they want to postpone having children. On the other
hand, they want children as their future security. To some extent, a
few of the teenage girls can afford to cohabit, i.e., live in a more informal marriage. Those who are economically empowered continue to
enjoy their economic independence and be able to take care of themselves.

One of the reasons for marriage is social prestige and to fulfil their
duties as responsible adult women. The young women think that
marriage is essential for their self-esteem and in order to conform to
the religious requirements and the values of society and to avoid
promiscuity. Some of them hope that marriage will entitle them to
some economic support.

Rozi from Songea explained why she had married: "When I
decided to marry, I thought that I would get financial assistance from
my partner. To my surprise, I am not getting any and my parents are
dead." Rozi was living with an unemployed man. Although she had
to use all her earnings to maintain herself, her husband, and their
child, Rozi still hopes that her husband will find some employment.
The girl still loves him. The man, however, does not show any interest
in formalizing their marriage in a Christian way.

From the interviews, it was clear that having children or being childless did not induce the teenage girls to marry. For those teenage girls who had experienced relationships with men, the wish to postpone marriage depended on their former experiences, such as being mistreated by their partners, or on their future plans of becoming economically secure and then finding a suitable partner.

For example, Kerubina, who has two children, says that she has no intent of marrying soon. In her own words: "I am saved and I am just serving our Lord. I don't wish to marry unless our Lord wishes so and gives me a good partner."

By a good partner she meant: one who is saved like herself and who will be able to take care of her children. Before she was saved she had a boyfriend by whom she bore the two children. This man had another wife. The man deserted her when her second born was only one month old. It was then that her life became difficult and Kerubina started to break and sell stones to be able to take care of herself and her children. She had been involved in her friendship with the man since she was 15 years old. At the time I met her she was 19.

Another girl, Ana, wants to marry as soon as the father of her two children agrees to marry her. She prefers to marry him because he is very kind to her. They get along very well. She would like stay together with him and plan the future of their children together. The only snag is that the partner has not yet proposed her.

Kasiana was married at 16 and divorced at 18. Her marriage had been arranged by her parents because her husband had many cows. Her father wanted bridewealth of ten cows. Moreover, her parents feared that if she was not married early, she might become promiscuous. Her husband treated her harshly, threatening to kill her. He was 55 years old and quite ruthless. He did not take care of his young wife. Kasiana's father did not want to return the cows. He, therefore, prevented the daughter from asking for divorce. Eventually, he allowed her to seek divorce after she threatened to kill herself. Kasiana does not want to remarry in the near future. She thinks all men are the same. She had one child by the man and she now takes care of the child. The father is not interested. He is married to another woman and preoccupied with the children of his other marriage.

The 18-year-old Fatu was obliged to marry her husband because their marriage was arranged by the parents on both sides. Her parents in particular wanted her to marry so that she did not become promiscuous. She was married off when she was only 15 years. Her husband was 40 years old. However, they are still living in harmony although the husband cannot meet all her needs. That is why she breaks stones.

Another girl thought that she had to marry because a woman cannot live without a husband. According to her, the only acceptable means of living with a man is through marriage. She herself chose her husband and she thinks that they love each other.

Maimuna had high hopes before she got married. She thought that after marriage her life would change for the better and that her husband would assist her economically. She has to support her parents who are old and sick. Before she got married she had no income. After they were married, her husband could not assist her. She, therefore, resorted to stone-breaking in order to earn some money to survive and to take care of her parents. After some time, their marriage began to fail. They divorced. Maimuna does not intend to remarry until she meets someone who can support her and her parents.

Work and family

Most of the teenage manual workers would like to have children during their lifetimes, irrespective of their marital status. Those who were married hold that four children is enough, while those who are not formally married considered two children as the maximum. Those who are still single think that children are important because they will take care of them in old age. The preferred number of children depends of their affordability, taking into consideration economic conditions. One girl said that the actual number of children depends on the will of God.

So far, the fifteen teenage workers in Songea have six children in total. In two cases, the mothers are only 16 years. The fifteen teenage workers in Dar es Salaam have five children in total. The two youngest mothers are 16 and 17 years respectively.

Those who have children but who are not married and are not cohabiting, do not want to increase the number of children unless they find a partner who will marry them and assist them with childrearing. Some of the married women postpone having children because they cannot do their manual work properly during pregnancy. However, there were others, who argued differently, like one of the Songea girls who was of the opinion that marriage and children improved her condition in that she has a mutual understanding with her husband about economic activities. The husband advises that she should not engage in brick-lifting all her life, and must devise a way out of this work. For the time being, she has not found an alternative.

The brick-lifters and stone-breakers observed that they cannot hire helpers for baby sitting, because it is very expensive for them. A few of them depended on their parents or the siblings they stay with to look after their young ones when they go to work on the construction sites or in the quarries.

For most of the stone-breaking mothers of Dar es Salaam, it was convenient to come to the site with their young ones, at to go back home quickly to take care of their housekeeping tasks such as cooking and washing. Most of them had hired rooms near their work site. For them, this job is much better than being employed in the formal sector, because with this job they can save the money which would otherwise be used for hiring a helper.

During my fieldwork, I observed some teenagers coming to work with their young children. In this way, their children are also taught the skills of stone-breaking. I found children ranging from one and above accompanying their mothers, the older ones helping by gathering stones and sometimes breaking them. One day, I saw a girl of 4 years using a hammer and breaking stones. I told her to stop, because I feared that the hammer could crush her fingers. To my surprise her mother, a 19-year-old worker, was watching her without any concern, implicitly encouraging her child to learn this skill. I came to learn later that the mother of the girl also had learnt the skill from her mother, who breaks and sells stones at the same site. She is the one who gave the investment capital to her daughter. On top of manual work, the stone-breakers are expected to support their husbands. When a husband is not employed, the wives have a heavier burden. If the husband is employed, he may share costs with her. Nevertheless, sometimes all the responsibility is left to the wife, even if the husband has a job.

The Songea brick-lifters work a good distance from places where they live, because their work depends on the location of the construction sites. For that reason, most of them leave their children with their parents, kin, or even neighbours. In some cases when they do not have anyone to look after their children, they resort to going to the sites with their children. It happened one day during my field work that Ostakia, a single mother of two, one of them still a small baby, decided to leave her baby at home without telling her mother that she was going to the site. Ostakia needed money. The father of the children was a security guard on one of the construction sites. Unfortunately, he had been dismissed from work, following the theft of some of the site's property, so he could not take care of her and the children. When the grandmother realised that Ostakia was nowhere to be seen, she followed her to the site with the baby in her arms and gave it to her daughter. Ostakia had to work with her baby tied on her back. Ostakia told that her mother too was desperately looking for a job. She had no husband who could take care of her. She sold porridge at the marketplace and could not do so with such a young baby in her care.

Most of the girls in the study thought that being pregnant, having young children, or being sick, could jeopardize their chances of gaining income by manual jobs. During advanced pregnancy and the first months after childbirth, or when sick, the brick-lifters and stone-breakers have to quit their occupations. During this time, they have to depend on the sympathy of their parents, kin, or their *wana ushirika*. Very few of them believe that they can manage on their own savings.

Conclusions

The teenage stone-breakers and brick-lifters come from a poor section of the rural population. They have been able to occupy jobs in the modern construction sector, jobs that do not seem to attract male workers or people in the urban community. However, there were examples of mothers who had introduced their daughters to the trade. Whereas people in general are not aware of women working in these relatively new fields, I did meet a few women who are second-generation stone-breakers. Given that workers live close to their worksites and that small children follow their mothers to work, it is to be anticipated that they start hammering stones in imitation of the adult women. I would not call it child labour; it looked more like keeping the children busy for awhile.

It appears that the quarries and construction sites mainly offer opportunities to unskilled migrant women. There are not many options for poorly educated rural teenagers. According to custom, men built the wooden structures and women plastered the mud houses, or they put mud between the bricks while the men built the roof of thatch or iron sheets. The men's part in house construction has also changed and the options for employment for rural migrant men are also restricted.

Some of the interviewed teenagers had relationships with men. These ranged from temporary to more permanent commitments, whether cohabitation or marriage. Marriage was considered an essential stage of life. Some teenagers expected that marriage would mean the sharing of costs with the husband, but found this was not always the case. The men they meet are also poor, their earnings are unreliable, the risk of unemployment high, so that they cannot live up to the girls' economic expectations. Many teenage girls have become more realistic. They break stones and lift bricks to supplement the meagre incomes obtained by their husbands. The unmarried girls often postpone marriages, and try to increase their own assets.

Being sick or pregnant or having children, sharing parental care or living as a single parent, these are all conditions which affect teenage girls in many ways. Being pregnant or breast feeding a child makes it hard to continue manual work. The networks of support were small and the means they commanded were limited. Most of the young girls had to resume their work before they had fully strength.

A comparison of the migrant teenage workers we studied in Songea and Dar es Salaam reveals some differences. The girls in Songea had more often finished primary school (7), while in Dar es Salaam more girls had married (9). The girls in Dar es Salaam were older (mostly 18 to 19 years) and had migrated over much longer distances. Moreover, in Dar es Salaam, the stone-breakers owned the stones and could thus set their own terms for selling their product, while in Songea the terms of pay were set by the owners of the buildings under construction. In addition, the teenage workers in Dar es Salaam live close to the worksite. This is a great advantage to them, because they can take care of their children and housework without seriously interrupting their stone-breaking. Contrariwise, in Songea the workers have to move to where buildings are being constructed at that time.

Nevertheless, in spite of differences, the stone-breakers and brick-lifters in Dar es Salaam and Songea have much in common. They face many health risks in the course of employment from the dust and cement which they inhale, from to the sun and the rain, from poor sanitary facilities, dirty drinking water, poor tools, and lack of protective gear. Because of their limited options, most of the girls are happy to have found a way to earn money. They work long days to improve their condition and hope to have children in a few years' time. However, they want no more than two to four children, whether they are married or not, because of their economic condition. Children are important, men are not to be trusted. Even so, many girls look for someone who will share responsibilities with them.

References

Boserup, E., 1970, *Women's Role in Economic Development*. London: Allen and Unwin.

Ebner, E., 1972, *The History of Wangoni*. Ndanda: Mission Press.

Epstein, C.F., 1970, *Women's Place, Options and Limits in Professional Careers*. Berkeley and Los Angeles: University of California, Press.

Hirchmann, D. and M. Vaughan, 1984, *Women Farmers of Malawi*. California: Institute of International Studies.

Manohar, K.U., 1984, *Socio-Economic Status of Indian Women*. New Delhi: Seewa.

Mnyagolo, R.B. et al., 1981, *Agizo la Mlale*. Ruvuma: Peramiho Printing Press.

Ntukula, M.N., 1990, *"Division of Labour and Sexual Inequality in Urban Tanzanian Households"*. Unpublished M.A. thesis, University of Dar es Salaam.

Rzhanista, L., 1983, *Female Labour under Socialism: The Socio Economic Aspects*. Moscow: Progress Publishers.

Standing, G.L., 1978, *Fertility and Female Labour Force Participation*. Geneva: ILO.

Stycos, J.N., 1964, *The Control of Human Fertility in Jamaica*. Ithaca: Cornell University Press, Ithaca.

Tanzania Demographic and Health Survey. Dar es Salaam: Bureau of Statistics, 1984.

Tanzania Knowledge Attitudes and Practice Survey. Dar es Salaam: Bureau of Statistics, 1995.

Chapter 9

Relationships for Survival
—Young Mothers and Street Youths

Virginia Bamurange

In my profession as counsellor, I have been exposed to much information about youth problems either directly through youths themselves
or through other professionals. As a result of this exposure, I decided
to study young mothers who had their firstborn out-of-wedlock and
of street youths. I have learned that, the most vulnerable youths, such
as unmarried teenage mothers and street youths, are often neglected
and rejected. Most of what I know about the worst off youths is what
other people think of them. I, therefore, developed a wish to find out
from teenage mothers and street youths themselves about their experiences and perceptions of their lives.

My second reason for undertaking this study arose from the facts
that I learned during an earlier study (Tumbo-Masabo and Liljeström,
1994), that dealt with expectant teenagers' and teenage mothers'
knowledge, attitudes and practices concerning reproductive health.
This work showed that teenage mothers mainly come from poor families and have had to leave school early. In Tanzania, the *Education Act*
requires pregnant girls to be expelled from school. None of the 120
girls we studied had learned sufficient skills to be able to earn an independent living.

In the above study, parents lamented the chaos that early pregnancy brought on their families, creating contention between parents
and adding to their economic burden. Undoubtedly, the teenage
mothers were biologically immature and economically dependent.
Moreover, they lived in an environment that was either hostile or in-
different to them. I kept asking myself, how do they raise their babies?
How do they cope with all the difficulties they face? What support, if
any, do they get from their communities?

I decided to revisit three of those teenagers and explore what had
happened to them. Do they earn a living on their own which enables
them to live and take care of their babies? Do they get any support

from their families and/or the fathers of the infants? I wanted to ascertain their feelings towards the child and to inquire about their prospects for the future.

Street youth is a category of youth which has always been a mystery to me. I have tried to puzzle out how these teenagers cope with street life while being so young, so poor, so unprotected, and so often hunted by the police. Efforts to help street youths have existed for a number of years, but their impact is still to be felt. There is glaring evidence that the number of street youths is increasing tremendously in Dar es Salaam. Therefore, it is worth knowing more about why they move on to the streets, how to assist them to make a living, and the vision they have for their future, before starting some kind of programme for them.

Thus, I decided to go out to the streets and make contact with some street adolescents. My aim was to explore their background, i.e., their families and education, and their lives before going on to the streets. I wanted to discover what attracted them to Dar es Salaam and how they earned their living. I also wanted to ascertain their experiences on the streets, their feelings about their situation, and their hopes for the future.

I met up with five boys and five girls, all of them "youths of the street", i.e., the street is their home where they seek shelter, a livelihood, and companionship. They may have occasional contact with their families. I chose to study this category of street youths because they are more vulnerable than the "youths on the streets", who engage in street-related trade, such as shoe-shining, but at the end of each day return to their families.

In the following section, I give an account of my follow-up with the three young mothers, their daily life of work, their relationships, and first and foremost, their relations with their child/ren. Thereafter, I guide the reader to the places in Dar es Salaam where street youths stay and share what I have found out about their strategies of survival.

Being a mother at the wrong moment

Kibibi

I had made my appointment with Kibibi through her grandmother. After discovering Kibibi's home, the first person I met was her grandmother, an elderly, well groomed lady who speaks fluent Kiswahili. She listened to me attentively, posed a few intelligent questions, and introduced me to Hawa, the lovely daughter of Kibibi.

Kibibi is now married to a businessman, but because of a housing problem she has moved in with her parents. The first day I met her, I was struck by her style of dress: she was very well dressed, looked confident and was responding very well to me. At the time of the previous study, she was 19 years old and had just started Form 3 in a girl's secondary school in Dar es Salaam when she fell pregnant. She was, of course, expelled. She narrated this to me without any sign of regret or remorse.

Kibibi is employed in a hair salon. She works there daily including Saturdays and Sundays, from 8:00 a.m. to 6:00 p.m. Mondays are free. She has one-and-half-hour lunch break. Her salary is used to buy clothes and food for her child. All her other costs are taken care of by her mother and Baba Mtoto, as she likes to call her husband.

I observed Kibibi's relationship with her child on Mondays, which is her day off when she can spend the day with her daughter. Even when she went visiting relatives and friends, her baby would go with her. The great-grandmother, lovingly known as Bibi Mkubwa, is, of course, always there, talking to both of them in a very friendly manner, advising and cautioning on almost every issue. She is very close to the child. The child behaves very differently with her. It was observed that Kibibi is a well trained mother. One can see that in the way she takes care to bath the child, cooking for her, and feeding her.

Kibibi told of her experience of motherhood. It had been rather hard when the child was still very young and had repeated attacks of malaria. She frequently went to hospital. Kibibi remembers that she was very worried, but as time passed, the child grew and became healthier. Kibibi also remembers the good times with the child. One could see how joyful Kibibi became. From the time the baby was 3 months, Kibibi used to play with her a lot. She liked to see her baby laugh and talk. But her biggest joy was when Hawa started to walk at the age of 9 months. She then started inviting other infants to play with Hawa and go with her for short walks. Kibibi is very satisfied with her life as it is now. She looked quite contented.

Little Hawa is very happy among the family members. She enjoys the attentive care showered on her by everybody, especially by her great-grandmother Bibi Mkubwa. She is spoilt. She can sit on Bibi

Mkubwa's lap, tell her infant stories, while Bibi Mkubwa listens attentively, corrects her, and plays with her. In another instant she is running errands for Bibi Mkubwa. Kibibi's siblings add to the joy of the child. She gets all their attention and she reciprocates with delighted looks.

Of her future plans, Kibibi told me with self-confidence that, "I have the skills to run a hair salon on my own. What I need is money, which I have started saving." She insists that before she has another baby, she would like to start her own hair salon.

Kibena

When I first met Kibena, it was at the prompting of a lady neighbour who saw her walking from a house after she had lied to the ten-cell leader and me that Kibena was her sister and not herself. The young mother looked very dirty. It seemed she had not washed her khangas, a traditional form of cloth, for a number of days. I used that first day just to establish a rapport with her. She invited me to her parent's home where she was staying and introduced me to her mother. There were a lot of toddlers and young children who belonged to her sisters. The children looked uncared for. The adults of the family always seemed to be away. In fact, the children took care of each other.

I had to meet her four times to conclude my interview, which I did with the other girls in a few hours. Kibena is shy, lies a lot, and doesn't have a good memory. With time and patience and appropriate questioning techniques, she talks and reveals a lot. I used many probes and prompts and examples to make her understand my questions. The way she expresses her emotions is scary. She can look very angry and then in a flash burst into loud laughter. One could easily conclude that she is unbalanced. Is she confused? Am I asking her questions nobody has asked her before? Am I giving her an opportunity to reflect on her life, to think deeper? Probably, she had never done that before and the feelings and insights are causing a strange reaction? Such thoughts crossed my mind whenever I was with her and by this means I was able to establish some empathy with her.

Kibena earns her living by selling vegetables. She leaves home early in the morning and goes to wait for the farmers on their way to sell their produce in Morogoro market. She buys a lot of cucumbers and comes back home at 9:00 a.m. She either sits at home lazily or goes visiting neighbours. The many toddlers and young children either play in the dust around the house or follow her on her visiting spree. They are all unwashed. She comes back at noon, prepares the cucumber (washing, slicing, and salting) and at 3:00 p.m. she sets out for the local bars to sell them. This is her daily routine and this is how she earns her living. Kibena comes back late at night from selling her cucumbers: most of the time she comes back drunk. She might easily fall pregnant again, for she has a number of escorts-cum-admirers. Kibena could not tell me what profit she makes, but at the end of the day she usually comes back with about 2,000 shillings (3 US dollars). The following day, she uses the balance to buy more cucumbers, but she also has to buy two kilos of *sembe* (maize flour) everyday to help support the family.

There is no way a stranger would know that Kibena has children. She does not interact with them at all. Her babies are intermingled with the children of her sisters. They all eat together. The older children take responsibility for the younger ones. The whole week I stayed in Morogoro, I spent an average of five hours there daily from morning till evening, accompanied by my research assistant. We never saw her playing, feeding, bathing, or doing anything with the children. No wonder she has no sense of attachment whatsoever to her children.

Talking of her experiences, Kibena said:

> When I had my first baby, I was 16 years old. It was a normal delivery. I was satisfied and my parents were satisfied too. My boyfriend came all the way from Dar es Salaam to see me. He is still helping me to raise the child. He gives me 3,000 shillings per month (about 5 US dollars) and he is going to take away his child very soon.

She uttered the last sentence with a sense of pride. I tried to explore on her feelings on some issues regarding motherhood, but Kibena expressed none. The repetition of "I was satisfied" in response to everything bored me. She didn't even remember with any special feeling the developmental stages of her babies. When she talked of the babies falling sick, she did not connect this with any feelings of worry, depression, or sadness. She would just say: "I used to take the baby to hospital."

The question of her future plans is the only one to which Kibena responds quickly, excitedly, and at any length. With bright eye she narrates and giggles:

After the father of my firstborn child takes him, which will be soon, I will look for a room to become independent. I will leave my second child here with my parents, because I do not want him to be lonely. He is used to living with a lot of people. I will have five more children. Of course, I will space them because I know I can get family planning services from UMATI. I am right now on the injection. I can do what I want and nothing will happen.

Asked whether she had plans to get married, she said, "It is not easy to get a man." Asked whether she could raise five children by herself, she responded, "My cucumber business will be enough."

Clara

It was not easy to trace Clara as she has no permanent place of abode. She sometimes lives with her parents, and at other times she is with her partner or the mother of her partner. I managed to conduct my study when she was with her partner.

The first day I saw her I was confused by her appearance. She still looks 14 years old, even after three years. One would think that she stopped growing after delivering her first baby. This might be biologically possible, for the nutrition that might have assisted her to grow was depleted by two pregnancies and by nursing two babies for she now had another baby. She is very timid, her face is blank, showing neither joy nor sadness. She evoked much concern in me.

Clara has two daughters, one is 3 years old and the other 5 months. She got her first baby when she was only 14 and was expelled from school. When she was attending an antenatal clinic at Temeke hospital, a nurse introduced her to the UMATI Young Mothers' Centre. She had a chance to complete her primary school at the centre and was selected to go to secondary school, which she never completed because of her second pregnancy. Clara gave this account in a very sad tone.

She is a housewife and is supported by her partner, who is employed. Her house chores include: cleaning the little room, laundry, washing dishes, bathing the baby, cooking for the baby, feeding the baby, and going to the market. "What I do from morning till evening is the same from Monday to Friday. It is very boring", says Clara.

Observation of the young mother's interaction with her daughter occurred in the quiet room where Clara lives with her partner. She performs one task after another in a very passive mood. After her partner leaves for his work at about 7:30 a.m., she cooks porridge for the child, bathes her, dresses her, and seats her on a mat on the floor. The child is not very quiet but there is no response from the mother. Is this her character or is she depressed? It is as if the child is served by a robot lacking the human touch! Then, to my surprise, she called somebody to take the baby away. On the first day I thought the baby would soon be brought back, so I waited for half an hour but the baby was not brought back. She had been taken to an old "mama's" house. The mama is given a token amount at the end of the month for taking care of the baby.

Clara has no permanent domicile. As an unmarried teenage mother, she has a semi-nomadic style of living. Such a situation has an effect on the psychological stability of any person. I wondered if this style of life was a survival strategy. Probably nobody was willing to stay with her on permanent terms, so she kept moving from her mother's house to her partner's and then to her partner's mother! It remained a riddle to me that such a person could be in a position to take care of a baby!

Upon my inquiring about her experience of motherhood, Clara's timidity and passivity broke. She talked regretfully, especially about the second pregnancy, which, she said, had robbed her of all the possibility of continuing school. It was as if this was the first time she had expressed her feelings about the situation, for she was overwhelmed by emotion, tears welling in her eyes, biting her lips, and lamenting: "Why did it happen again? Whatever was I thinking! I am not even happy with the choice of man I made. My family is unhappy too!" Ironically, Clara was prepared to marry the man the moment he suggested marriage! She does not know the whereabouts of the first man after he left her upon hearing news of the first pregnancy. She is not even sure if this second man will marry her.

Clara also shared with me her sad feelings about the whole episode. She angered her parents greatly, especially with her second pregnancy, "My parents were so angry that I was not allowed to live with them any longer", she said. Clara repeated the following statement three times during my interview, each time almost in tears: "I had two unplanned babies. They belong to two different men. This has compelled me not to live with my eldest daughter. She lives with my mother. I miss her and I am sure she misses my love. But my daughters are very sweet, and this gives me joy sometimes."

Nevertheless, she deprived herself of the opportunity of spending more time with her second daughter.

Clara was overcome by her sense of defeat. She is burdened by regrets: she was expelled from school, her parents do not want to live with her, her first partner ran away. The second has not promised marriage. This is too much for her. Her lack of real relationships in this difficult time is well illustrated in how she relates to her children. She is near to them, yet very distant. She does not respond to her baby's talk. She cannot handle a proper relationship because she has been failed by people around her.

Talking of her future plans, she says she is not satisfied with staying with a man without a formal marriage. Thus, her immediate concern for the future is to get married. It seems, however, that she continues to make decisions that are detrimental to her. She wants to marry a man who otherwise would not be her choice. I believe, she is complying with societal values and pressures at her own expense.

After marriage, she says she will look for a job or for training. She is interested in tailoring and her mother is already making arrangements for training.

The three young women as mothers

The three young women shared similar experiences of getting pregnant out-of-wedlock. Two were schoolgirls and one was an apprentice tailor. The two schoolgirls were expelled from school and the third had to leave her apprenticeship. After three years, the girls were found to be living different lives and having different aspirations. The social forces around them, i.e., their parents, their families, etc., had contributed much to the observed differences.

The life of Kibibi confirms that not all teenage mothers end in peril. Kibibi's experiences do not differ from those of any other mother who had a baby at more usual age after being married. To understand this situation, I had to visit her family and uncover this reality. By revisiting, I discovered that the parents of Kibibi had reacted differently from the norm in most Tanzanian tribal cultures. They were happy to learn that Kibibi was expecting. They may belong to an ethnic group where pregnancy before marriage is accepted, or they might have learned the news with sadness, but decided to support their daughter. Whatever the case, their response has worked well for all involved.

Contrariwise, my observation of Kibena's family and my talks with her make me feel that discouraging teenage pregnancy is like fighting a losing battle. Kibena seems detached emotionally from this important event in her life. She recounts her experiences with neither regret nor excitement. She does not relate to her two children. Neither does she cherish motherhood nor regret being an unmarried teenage mother. Her parents do not look upset either. She looks poor and her way of earning a living is precarious. She does not care. After all, her older sisters have done the same, and all the grandchildren are at their grandparents' home and nobody bothers with them. Why fuss? I could sense her thinking this as we spoke.

Yet, her future plans lack realism. She wants to be independent and have five more children. I do not envisage her raising five children on the basis of the petty business of selling cucumbers. Like many other adolescents, her decisions appear to be guided more by feeling than by reason. I ask myself how many other girls like Kibena do we have in our community and whether there is anybody there who can guide them and give them direction?

It was good to learn that Kibibi and Clara are convinced of the importance of having a few children and are already aware of methods of family planning and are practising them. They now know where to seek help. It is also encouraging to note that both girls want to be independent in future. If their wishes are supported with accurate information, and material, and moral support, the girls may not be caught in the vicious cycle of poverty. If they are supported by well considered interventions by their communities, things could improve for them. But does the society understand these obligations?

Mbunda (1990) examined whether traditional sociocultural controls affect adolescent premarital childbearing in Tanzania among the Wamatengo of Mbinga district, Ruvuma region. Mbunda concluded that the community did not know how to deal with this problem. When he interviewed parents and leaders on the means to contain it, 47 per cent confessed they did not know what to do, while 37 per cent thought a stern reprimand to their daughters would be enough. A similar community might surround Clara!

Relationships featured as a strong driving force in the lives of the young mothers, especially how the family members related to the girls during and after pregnancy. It seems that it was a failure of family relationships which put the lives of Kibena and Clara in peril. The young mothers have been affected by their family relationships and these relationships are mirrored in the way they relate to their own children as well as to themselves. Their ways of relating differed so much among each other, that one might think that I had chosen them as subjects for this very reason. This was not the case. Reflecting later on these relationships, I began to wish to see the children when they grow up. They will surely be very diːˤrent from each other. According to psychodynamic theories about the significance of the early childhood, these children will grow up presenting their pasts by showing different levels of trust, dependency, self-esteem, social skill, sexual identity, etc. (Jacob, 1993). Of course, Clara's and Kibena's children will be at a disadvantage according to these theories.

Street adolescents of Dar es Salaam

It has always been difficult for me to comprehend how a young boy or girl manages to survive on the streets. Yet, street boys and girls have been living and making money on the streets of Dar es Salaam for more than a decade now. Though their number to date has yet to be estimated, research conducted by the department of social welfare in February 1991 reported between 200 and 300 street children and youths in Dar es Salaam. Four years later, they are 3,500 (Saleh, 1995). These data evidence a tremendous increase. Indeed, anybody who has lived in Dar es Salaam for the past decade will have observed the proliferation of street children and youths.

My curiosity about how they survive led me to the streets to study their survival strategies, how they are exposed to sexual harassment, and how they, especially girls, use sexual services as means of survival. I also wanted to find out why they come to the city.

Why do they come to the city?

I met young Ndesario, my first subject, through a taxi driver in Dar es Salaam. The driver had seen me at the ferry fish market trying to get in touch with street boys. He took me to another site around Cameo cinema theatre in the early hours of the morning (about 6:00 a.m.). There I met Ndesario. I later learned that some street boys pay a token amount to cinema theatre/shop watchmen to sleep on the building verandahs.

After I had established a rapport with Ndesario, he became very instructive and an invaluable resource for my study. I learned from

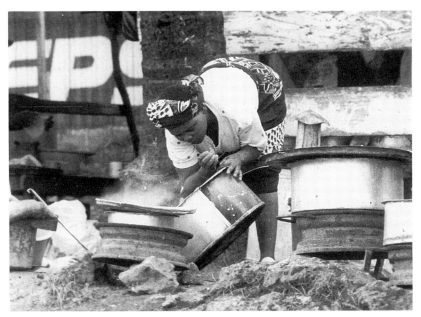

Mama ntilie are women who sell cooked food in the city.   (Photo Benny Kisanga)

him the other sites where I could find street youths and the appropriate time to approach them. This information was worth more than
that which I had gained from social workers during my initial
reconnaissance.

Ndesario claims to have been born in northern Tanzania, in the
Kilimanjaro region, about 600 kilometres from Dar es Salaam.

> My parents were peasants. When I was young, my father died and my
> mother remarried immediately. My mother told me that I was to be
> raised by my grandfather, who was a widower. But my grandfather, un-
> able to maintain me, sent me away, saying that it was my mother who
> should bear the responsibility. My mother refused and I became tired of
> shuttling from one house to another with the message of my rejection, so
> I ran away. My friends had told me that in Moshi you could easily get
> money, so I worked and lived on the streets there for sometime before
> coming to Dar es Salaam.

Ndesario remembers with amusement how, when he was still in his
home village, he made friendship with a bus conductor by doing his
laundry and keeping him company. After awhile, he pleaded with the
bus conductor to give him a free ride because he did not have the
money for a fare.

Ndesario survives on the streets by doing all sorts of odd jobs. He was observed picking over articles from the then Kisutu dump. These articles ranged from charcoal to empty cans of beer, that can be sold for recycling. Ndesario gathers anything that can be sold: "One never knows what one can get for garbage. I once found a torch which I sold for 5 000 shillings" (about 8 US dollars). A person like Ndesario could buy twenty meals with that amount or get a pair of jeans and a T-shirt from a secondhand clothstore commonly known as a *"mitumba"*.

Charcoal is lucrative for the boys. It is sold in small bags to *mama ntilie* at 250 shillings per bag. *Mama ntilie* are women who sell cooked food in the city. For 250 shillings one can buy a plate of rice and beans or vegetables from her. On a good day, Ndesario can sell two or three bags of charcoal. Ndesario has never been to school. He can neither read nor write, but when I inquired how he could count his money, he laughed and said "As a man I must know how to count money."

I learned from Ndesario that relationships with people around him are very important in his life on the streets. Little Ndesario, who does not look more than 13 years old explained to me that "One has to be very careful in choosing a group to belong to for one needs to conform to the norms and habits of the group. Before you decide to join, you test the situation. When you are satisfied that you can meet their norms, then you show your total allegiance to the group."

I met my second subject, Ndolela, at the Kisutu dumping ground under the guidance of Ndesario. When I went there, I found several boys lying on the ground covered by their jackets on the verge of the dump. It was about 6:00 a.m. I observed that the older boys guarded the younger ones. Ndesario pointed to a place and said "Ndolela is sleeping over there." He cautioned me: "We cannot approach him if that older boy sitting with him does not agree. We should talk to him first." The older boy, who looked to be very much in charge and full of pride, was approached, but rejected our request claiming that Ndolela was still tired. This suggested a caring relationship. We made an appointment and I was able to see Ndolela the following day. We did not spend much time in cultivating confidence. The laughing, chubby Ndolela told me that he trusts whatever Ndesario tells him and that Ndesario had told him I was a good mama. Ndesario told me that the older boy is from Ndesario's home area.

The 15-year-old boy hails from Mtwara, about 400 kilometres from Dar es Salaam. He had come to the city by bus. He went to school for four years and can read and write. He looks a healthy, strong boy. The reason for his coming to the city is family problems. "After my mother was divorced, my father remarried and of all the children I was the one who did not get on well with my stepmother. My father sent me to live with my aunt. I did not like her, so I ran away."

I also came to know a boy called Maasai, because of his typically Maasai looks. I met him near the Motel Agip area late in the evening. This tall majestic boy was giving orders to the others and he seemed to command respect. I later learned that he is a veteran in the area. Maasai and the other boys were busy guiding car owners into parking areas. These people had come for an evening out at Motel Agip restaurant.

The Maasai boy hails from Morogoro, 200 kilometres away. He had been in the city for three years. His main goal was to work for money to help his mother raise his three other brothers. His father had died of cancer. He earned the money by washing cars, guiding cars into parking lots, and guarding cars in one of the smart areas of Dar es Salaam. He earns 1,500–2,000 shillings on a good day.

He no longer sleeps outside like the other boys, but in the buses that are parked around Motel Agip area overnight. He is able to do this because of his relationship with the watchman of the area.

I found Mugisha, a 16-year-old boy, at a parking lot where Mkwepu Street and Mansfield cross. He comes from Kagera, a district 1,800 kilometres from Dar es Salaam. Like the other boys, he used public transport to reach the city. This timid sickly boy shared with me his background:

"We are a family of five. My father abandoned us and married a younger wife. They went to live in another town. I came here to earn money for my mother to bring up my sister and brothers." He earns money by washing cars and guarding parked cars along Mansfield Street.

Mugisha had left home to make money and to start a small business to help his siblings. Mugisha had worked hard for one year but had not realized his goal. He was prepared to tolerate another year on the street.

When I first met Bhoke on Mkwepu Street, I wanted to enlist his aid to find a street boy in that area. There is no way his personality reveals that he is a street boy. He is tall and clean and was sitting on the pavement outside a closed shop. He was solemnly reading an English magazine. I greeted him, he stood up and respectfully responded *"Shikamoo"* as is expected in this society from a young person. I expressed my wish to enlist his aid. He listened to me attentively, took time to observe me, and then replied slowly and clearly, "I am one mama!" I must have shown astonishment, for he repeated "I am a street boy mama. I work on this street and live on the streets."

The 19-year-old Bhoke comes from Musoma, 1,900 kilometres away. He told me that on a good day he fetches 1,500–2,000 shillings, which is what a skilled official earns in Tanzania. Washing a car is 200 to 300 shillings, while guarding a car is 200 to 599 shillings, depending on the time of the day and the length of time. "When I am lucky, I get three to five cars a day", says Bhoke.

Other jobs done by streets boys at specific times include carrying passengers' luggage at bus terminals and carrying packages of newspapers to bus stops. Bhoke has done this several times in the early hours of the day before buses leave the main bus stand for upcountry regions.

Regarding on what brought him to the city, Bhoke serenely recounts, "After I lost both my parents, we had a lot of disputes in the family. I decided to come here to search for a job. I had saved 3,000 shillings but it was too meagre to pay my fare, so I made friends with the bus conductor and I would run errands for him. In return, he gave me a free ride."

All the street youths I met had similar stories to tell. I found that they all used public transport to travel to the city from their home villages. Having insufficient money for fares, they depended on the goodwill of bus conductors with whom they had cultivated friendships. In order to cope with their daily lives, they learn such skills as establishing relationships and developing them into permanent links. Other adolescents in normal situations do not usually form permanent links and are usually cautious about the strong emotions that accompany the maintenance of relationships.

Relationships for survival

Relationships with significant people living and working near the street youths helps them survive the hardships of street life. Indeed, adolescents on the streets negotiate for their most lost basic rights with the people around them.

It has been found that for street youths earning a living on the street is a process that is new to them, uninformed and poor as they are. Gradually, after forging relationships and getting to know the city well, a dirty boy will shift to a cleaner job with more pay. This was true of the five boys I studied. The more recent arrivals are at the garbage dump in Kisutu. They looked dirty, insecure, and poor. Those who have spent two or more years on the streets were found near the smarter areas of Dar es Salaam. They looked cleaner, more confident and better organized.

The veterans were found to be near smarter centres or hotels such as the Mkwepu/Mansfield area and Motel Agip washing and guarding cars. In busy streets such as Samora Avenue, they assist drivers to park their cars. It is worth noting that in other parts of the world, street youths engage in similar activities. Kenosi (1991) writes about the tasks the street youths in Gaborone engage in, namely, car washing, grocery carrying, and car parking.

Creating and maintaining relationships is of great value to existence on the street. I observed this very early in my research. As I was searching for the subjects, I found that street youths are well organized regarding caring, protective, and trusting relationships with each other. After my pilot survey, I was more convinced that the fish market at Magogoni ferry would be a good area to meet street youths. I knew that these youths remain around fish merchants, ready to clean fish, run errands, and clean tables for money etc. I was flabbergasted when these merchants completely refused to let me talk to the boys, refusing even to disclose that the boys were street boys. Instead they told me that the boys were their sons. I concluded that the relationships had been cemented and that the boys were being closely protected.

All the boys in my sample were adolescents. Normally adolescents easily cause trouble in relationships, being guided as they are more by emotion than wisdom. This is to be expected, for adolescence is the time when teenagers seek self-identity and lack experience of life. This situation usually makes them vulnerable in establishing relationships. One could say that circumstances have forced these street boys to grow beyond their years. Indeed, the five boys shared with me that these relationships are about belonging, acceptance, protection, and most of all, about important information needed to survive street life.

Mama ntilies

Mama ntilies are women who sell cheap cooked food on the streets. Ndesario sells charcoal to *mama ntilies* for cash, or for credit against the day when he fails to make money and needs a plate of rice and vegetables. Sometimes he washes dishes or fetches water for a plate of food. "It is easy in this city not to go on an empty stomach, if you are clever enough", he told me. I heard the same tale from other boys.

Mama ntilies protect the boys from the police by claiming that they are their sons. Also, at the ferry fish market the fish merchants claimed that the boys were their sons who helped them with their trade and that whoever said that they were street boys was a liar.

Kiosk vendors

After I had gained their trust, the boys used to boast about the amount of money they had saved. My dilemma was to understand how they can save, and so many questions crossed my mind. They live on the streets, so where do they keep their money? The boys shared with me that they save money for a long-term goal, which for most of them is to help their widowed or divorced mothers and their siblings. Indeed, Mdogo had saved 20,000 shillings (about 30 US dollars) after eight months and has bought clothes for his sister and visited her in Lusotho about 100 kilometres away. He also had managed to move her to their aunt's home in Tanga. Maasai had saved 30,000 shillings (40 US dollars) and given it to his mother to start a petty business.

One day Maasai confided in me: "We save our money with the kiosk vendors." In my ignorance, I asked him about the precautions they take. Do they have witnesses? Do they have written and signed agreements? The boy was amused by my naiveté! He told me:

> All those written things do not make sense to us, for most of us do not know how to read or write. Moreover, if a person is not our friend, even if you write a million papers, he will still play tricks. We depend on the friendships we create with them. One has to be very careful: you do not just go to any kiosk vendor. You first explore which of them can be trusted. We use our brains. After you create a relationship, after the trust is there, he knows you well and you know him or her and you have created a sort of a bond based on likeness and trust. You sell the idea to him or her. You do not use force. In most cases they agree.

This arrangement is also beneficial to the kiosk vendor, for he continues to work with the money and does not pay interest. Thus the kiosk vendor also benefits from what little money is available. I later learned that the street boys commonly use kiosk vendors to save their money and none had ever been disappointed by them.

Maasai took me to his "banker" nearby his workplace and asked proudly how much he had saved. The kiosk vendor replied politely, 30,000 shillings (equivalent to 50 US dollars), enough to start a petty business in Tanzania. The boy searched seriously in his pocket notebook so to confirm this information. I was astonished! In a big city like Dar es Salaam most people cannot be trusted. One cannot entrust money to anybody. There must be signatures and witnesses, etc. The boy told me he has never written a contract but relies on his trusting friendship with the kiosk vendor.

Babus (watchmen)

The watchmen of the big buildings in the city, popularly known as *babus*, which means grandfathers, offer the street youth places to sleep. The street adolescents pay for the service, thereby enabling the watchmen to supplement their meagre incomes by night. The street adolescents also gain by being protected from rain, police, and people who might abuse them sexually.

So far I have emphasized supportive relationships built on trust and mutual assistance. It is a rather positive and encouraging picture. Unfortunately, it is not the whole truth. There is an other story to be told, a story of fear, abuse, petty crime, exploitation, and neglect.

Relationships of exchange and exploitation

Their boys' ability to budget their earnings is also surprising, given their level of literacy and their youth. In the course of this study, I was interested to explore what they do when all else fails. One said:

"It is very easy, I wash dishes for *mama ntilie* and get a plate of food." Another said that when he realizes that it was about four o'clock in the afternoon and he has not got anything to eat, he resorts to begging. Still another said he eats with his fellows. No illegal activity was reported. I observed that when Ndesario did not have any food before three o'clock, he yawned and dosed and then started for the ferry fish market where he was seen visiting Sodoma and Gomorrah. This seems to be an area for homosexuals. Was Ndesario going to give into homosexuality for money, I asked myself?

Street boys of all ages talk about sexual exploitation as one major problem they face. The boys feel humiliated and ashamed. Most boys avoid admitting that it has ever happened to them but clues and hints were given. Some boys admitted that "it happens to everybody when they are still young and new to the streets."

Some boys told of men who come to the Kariakoo market in vehicles loaded with grain, vegetables, and fruits from upcountry regions. These men have to wait with the vehicles for two or three days before going back to their regions. The boys call them goods carriers. They spend their time at Kariakoo market on the pavements and sleep there as well. Some young street boys also spend nights in this place. The goods carriers make friends with the boys who are so inexperienced that they do not yet have any way to earn money. A boy is bribed with a plate of food by the goods carrier and is then forced to spend a night with him being sodomized.

In addition, some of the veteran street boys, or as they are commonly known by other street youths, *watemi* or *wababe*, i.e., the chiefs or the powerful, were also identified as sexual exploiters of the younger and the newer boys. Julian, now 21, remembered his early days on the streets:

> When we became used to the city, we started sleeping in different places, including around cinema halls like the Cameo and the Odeon. We were by then more afraid of the *watemis* than the police. For when they found you, they could not only sodomize you but also steal all the money you had in your pockets.

Christopher, now 22, explained:

> Life in the beginning was a mixture of excitement and fear. We used to clean fish at ferry fish market and earn money to buy our meals. In the evening, we would set out to look for a place to sleep. We, the younger boys, were at risk of being sexually abused by the *watemi*. The *watemi* used to get the younger boys and force them to go to the golf grounds where various sins were committed.

This was confirmed by Mdogo, who had been in the streets for four years.

> When one is young and still new, the *watemi* hunt for your sleeping place and force you to the Gymkhana golf grounds and sodomize you. They are so many that you are left nursing your wounds. So we used to

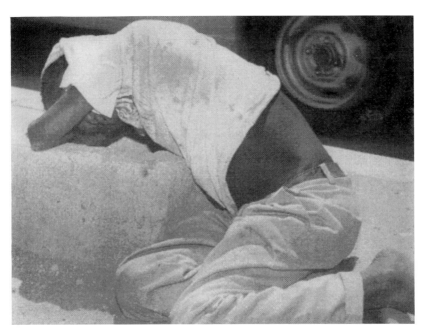

A street boy having a nap.   (*Pressphoto*, Dar es Salaam)

gang up in small groups of the same age and sleep near the streets where
the police patrol and at the same time hide from police, because they
used to take us to Central Police Station and arrange for our return home.
In our hiding places, whenever we saw *watemi* approaching, we would
cry out "police". The police used to save us.

On the wrong side of the law

Ndolela was once caught by the police when he was pick-pocketing in
a city bus, *daladala*, heading for Ubungo. No wonder street boys are
commonly known in Dar es Salaam as thieves. Mugisha, too, was one
day caught by the police for pick-pocketing. These young boys are
also paid to scout for bigger boys. This information was obtained from
an older boy who claimed not to involve himself in illegal activities.
Scouting for bigger boys means going to various assigned areas and
reconnoitring what people possess that can be stolen and sold. They
also determine the appropriate time to break in, etc. The five boys like
to boast of living a decent life despite what people think of them. I still
feel that they resort to stealing and other bad behaviour when their
meagre resources fail them.

All five admitted that life had not been easy. Besides the permanent fear one has of being caught by the police, there are also feelings of insecurity, of not knowing how you will earn your living, of falling prey to bad boys, of falling sick, and of dying so far away from one's family.

Deals for protection

Since earning opportunities are unequal between adolescent boys and girls, street girls mainly provide sexual services as a strategy of survival, while boys, as we have seen, have been able to improvize several income earning activities, even a kind of career, on the dumping grounds and by serving car owners at hotel areas. The girls' careers depend on men who are willing to pay for them.

Aisha, Julita and the other girls

When I met Aisha in 1995, she was 16 years and had been on the streets for seven years. She comes from a remote village in Tanga region in the east. Her parents divorced when she was about 7. Her mother remarried soon after and her father lived and worked in Dar es Salaam. The little girl was taken to live with her old granny. The granny was so old and frail that Aisha was the one taking care of her. Aisha felt this as a burden and negotiated with a bus conductor who knew her father to give her a lift to Dar es Salaam so that she could join her father. But her father was an alcoholic. He used to come home drunk after midnight. Then he would be violent. Therefore, Aisha used to go out at night and soon she struck up a relationship with some street girls. After awhile, she started spending the whole night out and it did not take long before she spent all her time on the streets.

Aisha was only 9 when she started fending for herself on the streets. She joined a small group of other girls. They survived by cooking for some street boys who used to bring them food. The cooking was done at *Mwembeni,* under a big mango tree at the ferry fish market.

> We used to spend daytime in abandoned boats for fear of the police. At night, we would all go to sleep on the enclosed verandah of a large shop in the city. We paid *babu* a token amount for this service. The boys used to protect me then, but when I reached puberty and my body began to change, they all wanted me for sex. This is the plight of most street girls. I

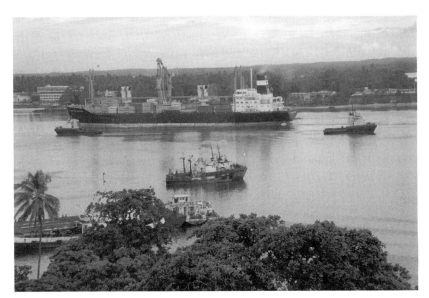

The girls spent the day on an abandoned boat.   (Photo Rita Liljeström)

had to run away. A fish merchant with a home in Kinondoni saved me from the monsters. Since then, we have been lovers and he provides me with lunch everyday, money for clothing, a place to rest during the day when his parents are not home. He has told me that he will never marry me but I cannot leave him unless I get somebody else who will support me.

It is worth noting that the relationship Aisha built with other girls and with the *babu* enabled her to survive street life. Her relationship with the fish merchant is also for survival as is clearly indicated in her account. Aisha is not the only girl who has a semi-permanent relationship.

Julita, 17 years, looked very happy and successful in her own way. She was well dressed in new clothes compared to the other girls, who wore secondhand clothes, and she was envied by them. The source of this envy is her rich lover who owns a shop in the city centre. Julita meets her lover everyday in his shop. There is a bedroom and a shower. Julita gets all her provisions from the shopkeeper. She spends her nights with the other girls on the verandah of a shop where they pay the *babu* a token amount. Her boyfriend collects her every night from the *babu's* place and spends some hours with her. Though he has forbidden her to greet him in public or show any recognition of him and told her, that she should not loiter near his shop, Julita seems satisfied with the relationship.

Julita and Aisha sleep at the *babu's* place with another eighteen girls. They did not reveal the name of the shop for fear that the *babu* would be caught and the service would come to en end. They pay 50 to 100 shillings each to the *babu*. For a whole month, the *babu* can earn the equivalent of his salary or almost double it. This is a good deal. The watchman will make sure that he safeguards this relationship and maintains it.

Protection of motherhood

I encountered the poorer girls on the streets under a big tree in an area known as Mkunguni, opposite the Tanzania Front Lutheran church. It is located along a beach. The girls spent the day on an abandoned boat, cooking the little food they had managed to buy, and resting after their long night hours on the streets. They looked undernourished and very poor. Of the group of twelve, two girls had babies. The relationship the girls had developed with Asia, a mother of a one-and-a-half-year-old son, deserves mentioning. The girls confided that they survive by prostitution. But as young and poor as they are, they have forbidden Asia, who is breastfeeding her child, to go on the streets. Instead, they share with her whatever they get. They all contribute to feed the baby. One day, Asia went on the street. Afterwards she received a good beating, and she promised the girls never to repeat the mistake. The girls were protecting the mother and the baby, and they were abiding by traditional norms whereby a breastfeeding mother abstains from sexual intercourse. According to various myths and beliefs, male semen pollutes the breast milk, so that the child will be affected by illness or weak growth. Such beliefs and their observance by female age-groups traditionally affected the spacing of children. In this way, people in polygamous marriages but without scientific knowledge about reproduction successfully spaced their children.

Babus, the grandfatherly pimps

Asia and her friend Aminata explained their street lives to me. Again, the story of *babus*, the watchmen, arose. The girls earn their living by prostitution. They go to the streets at night. The *babus* act as the go-betweens for the men who want the girls and provide a place where for them to meet. Asia and Aminata admit that it is hard to compete with sophisticated commercial sex workers, who are all along the street at night in smart clothes, wearing perfume and make up, and talking some English. "So we have to depend on the *babus*", they confided. The men pay these *babus* after each visit. The whole cycle is a relationship among vulnerable people who use each other for gain. The poor watchman use the poor girls of the streets and probably even the men who consort with these girls are poor. They cannot afford "sophisticated prostitutes". This type of relationship based on exchange and interwoven with dependency is well understood and managed by all those who participate in it.

Street girls were also exploited by several of the *babus* who provided sleeping places and male clients for the girls. Unlike the boys, the girls do not realize that they are being exploited. For example, Vumi, whom I first met at Mnazi Mmoja in a public TV place, looked very young and poor. She had run away from her stern stepmother in Iringa. In Dar es Salaam, she was selling sexual favours to get food. She was sleeping with other girls at one of the big markets. When she has a man, the market watchman allows them to use a corner of the market if they pay him. She told me that the same watchman also gets sexual favours from her. "He used to fondle me when I had a flat chest. But as my breast grew, we had the real act. This is my payment for sleeping at the market place." This *babu* gets paid twice! The men pay him as well. How many Vumis are there on the streets? This is exploitation, but this did not register in Vumi's young mind.

Relationships for survival and death

Teenage motherhood has been a great concern in the country for more than two decades now. Programmes have been initiated to combat the problem but the dilemma and the struggle continue. It remains a fact that teenage pregnancy and motherhood is a problem to the individuals concerned, their families, and the community at large. Intervention programmes should, therefore, aim not only at individuals but also at their families and the communities. The above study of three mothers shows that significant persons around them continue to influence their behaviour and their direction in life. I strongly recommend the identification and consideration of such forces before initiating intervention programmes.

The narratives of street adolescents about what moved them to come to Dar es Salaam provide glaring evidence of the failures of family relationships. The plight of these young people who shoulder family responsibilities when their parents die or are incapacitated, leaves one wondering about what has happened to the good African family structures that used to care for such people. The poor boys have been failed by their families and by their communities. Where are their uncles, aunts, etc.? In other instances, the role of parents has been reversed such that it is now the children who take care of the parents. To aggravate the situation, there are no alternative institutions in the communities to compensate for the absence of functional families.

Indeed, the above situation does not differ much from what is happening in other parts of the world. My study shows how adolescents create relationships that facilitate survival, how they are victimized, and drawn into life-threatening relationships. Sex has never been more threatening to health than it is today. This is because of HIV/AIDS. Sex is even more dangerous for this type of adolescent who is poor, unprotected, uninformed, and unguided. I am convinced there is a high probability that they will test HIV positive. The sexual abuse and exploitation of street adolescents is a strong indication of sexual illhealth. Probably they also suffer from sexually transmitted diseases without getting treatment. It is time that intervention programmes incorporated sexual and reproductive health services if they are to help adolescents in a holistic way. The paramount need for guidance, counselling, and shelter at nights cannot be overemphasized.

When I asked the youths about their future plans, they all had the same refrain: "To earn enough money and settle somewhere into Tanzania into a decent life." Will they manage?

Two years have elapsed since I conducted my interviews. I no longer see the serene Bhoke. His friends informed me that he got enough money to go home. Are they all as successful in realizing their goals? This is yet unknown! Eight months ago I met Maasai. He looked thin and had a rash all over his body. He told me that he had been in prison for six months. "Yes, the police finally got me, mama. I was sleeping in a bus. I had paid the watchman. In the middle of the night they stormed the bus and since I did not have any identity card and couldn't tell my proper address, etc. I was arrested." Now he was back, ready to work on the streets again.

It is hard to comprehend how street youths survive their poverty that verges on starvation, their exposure to the risk of diseases, their unhygienic work environment, their lack of shelter, their exposure to tropical rain and the malarial mosquitoes of Dar es Salaam. And they are always being hunted by the police!

From the little I shared with the street adolescents, I remain convinced that their struggle represents that of many other street youths. I would no longer label them dirty, and ill-behaved as I used to, but see them as victims of eroding communal obligations including taking care of each other and ensuring that members of the community fulfil their responsibilities—obligations that are no longer practised. This erosion, coupled with the economic hardship imposed by global policies such as Structural Adjustment Programmes, has prevented parents from coping with the plight of their children, who are robbed of their childhood and youth.

There is still hope of remedying this situation if we pool our resources, and apply well-resourced teamwork to helping these youths where they are—on the streets.

References

Arimpoor, J., 1992, *Street Children of Madras. A Situational Analysis*. National Labour Institute.

Black, M., 1991, *Philippines: Children of the Runaway Cities*. Florence: UNICEF.

Centres for Population Options, 1990, "Out of the Shadows. Building an Agenda and Strategies for Preventing HIV Infection and AIDS among Street and Homeless Youths". Conference report, May 1989.

Espinola, B., B. Glauser, R.M. Ortiz, S.O. de Carrizosa, 1988, *Asuncion—A book for Action*. Bogota: UNICEF.

Jacob, M., 1993, *The Presenting Past. An Introduction to Practical Psychodynamic Counselling*. London: Butler and Tanner.

Kainamula, V.B., 1994, *Survival Strategies of Teenagers*. Stockholm: Research Report to SAREC.

Kenosi, G.I., 1991, "Drug Abuse: Rehabilitation Programmes for Street Children in Botswana". Unpublished paper presented at the 4th International Symposium on Mobile Youth Work. Stuttgart.

Manumba, R.G., 1996. "The Situation of Street Children within the Legal System: Police Experience with Street Children". (Unpublished.)

Mbunda, W., 1990, "The Power of Extended Family, Social and Cultural Controls on Adolescent Pre-marital Childbearing among Wamatengo of Mbinga District, Tanzania". M.A. dissertation. (Unpublished.)

Mwakyajala, T.E., 1993 , "Problems and Dilemmas of Street Children in Tanzania: A Case Study of Dar es Salaam Region". Unpublished M.A. dissertation, Institute of Development Studies, Dar es Salaam University.

—1996, *Alcohol and Drug Abuse among Street Children in Tanzania. The Case of Dar es Salaam Region.* Research report for ADIC.

Rajan, R. and M. Kudrati, 1994, *Street Children of Mwanza. A Situation Analysis.* Kuleana.

Saleh, A.H., 1995, *The Street Children of Dares Salaam.* Report for DANTAN.

Rugumyamheto, A., V. Kainamula and J. Mziray, 1994, "Adolescent Mothers" in Z. Tumbo-Masabo and R. Liljeström, (eds.), *Chelewa, Chelewa. The Dilemma of Teenage Girls.* Uppsala: Scandinavian Institute of African Studies.

Chapter 10
Pregnancy Is Not the End of Education

Alice K. Rugumyamheto

> *I have been expelled from school. My parents are very poor, my boyfriend has no income. We definitely cannot bring up the child when it is born. My relatives and friends cannot help me either. My parents are very strict. They won't stand it when they learn I am pregnant. They will chase me from home. I must get rid of it. I have to get away from this shame. I will take fifteen chloroquine tablets and then complain of malaria. I know it is illegal but I have to do it. God will forgive me.*
>
> (Amina, a 17-year-old, Form 3, soon after learning that she was pregnant)

After overdosing on tablets she was rushed to the hospital unconscious. The hospital is about forty kilometres away. After examining the girl, the doctor discovered that she was pregnant and that she had attempted an abortion. By then it was too late and the doctors could do nothing to save her. She died two hours after being admitted to the hospital.

This is a true story about a girl who lived in my village. The incident prompted me to conduct a study of training institutions available to unmarried teenage mothers. The idea of training those young mothers appeals to me because it serves as an alternative which gives hope in place of the desperation that can claim a teenage mother's life.

In Tanzania, schoolgirls who fall pregnant are not allowed to continue their studies no matter how bright in class they may have been. These young mothers face a lot of limitations which hinder them from becoming useful members in the society. The foremost limitation is the fact that they lack training and, therefore, cannot be easily absorbed into the labour market or become self-employed. Second, most teenage mothers do not know of the existence of suitable training centres. Some teenage mothers get so frustrated and demoralized by their fate that they loose their self-esteem and confidence. The duty of taking care of the baby is another limitation, unless her parents are willing to assist while their daughter is undergoing training.

A recent study (Rugumyamheto et al., 1994) showed that parents of teenage mothers are compelled to take care of both their daughter and her child, since most of the young mothers are not financially independent. In most cases, parents are reluctant to let their daughters have any training after pregnancy because they fear that she might conceive again. Most teenage mothers just sit back waiting for the chance to get married but in our society once a girl falls pregnant out-of-wedlock, her chances of marriage are limited.

The formal education system has a number of post-primary vocational institutions such as the Folk Development Colleges (FDC) and National Vocational Training Centres (NVTC) which provide vocational training to young mothers. Most parents, however, cannot afford to pay the tuition.

Recently in Tanzania, some non-governmental organizations (NGOs) have established training centres to provide for girls who have dropped out of school due to pregnancy or who have completed primary education but became pregnant before acquiring any vocational skills. Such training centres are found in Dar es Salaam, Iringa, Songea, and Mbeya.

I decided to visit three of these institutions to learn how they are run, the curriculum offered, and whether it is relevant to the girls. I also wanted to know the objectives in establishing these centres and their backgrounds. Furthermore, I wanted to explore the problems these institutions face by having students who are mothers, and the attitudes of the parents towards educating their daughters.

To gain some first impressions, I undertook a pilot project by visiting the Temek Youth Centre in Dar es Salaam. The centre was established by the Family Planning Association of Tanzania (UMATI). I soon realized that my study was sensitive because it evoked the emotions of the teenage mothers. The management of the institution was also rather defensive, as such centres are still a new development in Tanzania. That is why so many people are interested in studying and visiting the Temeke Centre.

The main objectives in establishing training institutions for unmarried teenage mothers were: to enable girls who drop out of school at an early age to continue with their education; to provide knowledge and skills which will enable the teenage mothers to become self-reliant and raise their children; and to demonstrate to government and the general public that teenage mothers can be useful members of the society. An added objective is to discourage abortion among schoolgirls by offering them an alternative.

In the end, I visited three training centres, Matumaini Centre in Iringa, the Mama Clementina Foundation at Weru Weru Secondary School in Moshi, and the UMATI Youth Centre in Mbeya.

Matumaini Centre

The centre was started in 1990 by the Maryknoll Sisters in Iringa. Funds to run the centre are obtained from the Maryknoll Sisters, donors such as the Nordic Congregation, charitable donations, fund-raising activities, and self-reliance projects like a vegetable garden, and poultry and piggery projects. During my familiarization visit, the head of the centre had this to say to me: "We decided to work particularly with adolescent mothers in Tanzania after establishing that this group has been neglected by society. We realized that although most of them fall pregnant through ignorance about reproductive issues, society is normally unsympathetic towards them."

While visiting the centre for the first time, I saw a large poster at the entrance announcing the *Matumaini Youth Centre*. When I inquired about the name, one of the teachers said that the name *Matumaini* was chosen to portray hope, since this is how the word can be literally translated from Kiswahili into English. "We felt that the teenage mothers need to be given some hope in life. We wanted to show them that despite pregnancy they could still advance themselves educationally even up to university level, provided they had the necessary determination."

Teenage mothers are scattered and there is no structured system which deals with them. I wanted to establish how the girls gain admission. One of the teachers explained: As soon as the centre was ready we started looking for teenage mothers. To begin with, I contacted the ward executive officers and gave out flyers which I had prepared. The flyers stated: "Girls who got pregnant at school or at home are welcome to join a training centre at Saba Saba Iringa town." After a week I learned that no one had responded to the flyer. The ward executive officer told me that the poor response was due to the way the flyer was written. I decided to change the wording of the flyers. The new advert read: *A training centre has been opened at Saba Saba for young women who would like to advance themselves educationally*. The response was quite encouraging. Within a week, we received more than fifty applicants. However, we decided to admit only twenty-seven."

The head of the centre, a Maryknoll sister, is assisted by two full-time teachers, as well as four part-time teachers who are from a nearby secondary school, to fill in gaps in the coverage. A number of subjects are offered: bookkeeping, agriculture, mathematics, history, geography, needle-work, cookery, Kiswahili, biology, physics, chemistry, family life and health education, and legal affairs and women's rights.

School begins at 8:00 a.m. and ends at 3:00 p.m. Core subjects are taught in the morning while secondary school subjects are normally taught in the afternoon. Traditional dance is offered once a week as an extracurriculum activity.

However, teaching materials are inadequate. There are no laboratories so students are forced to concentrate on theory at the expense of traditional science subjects. There is a library for general reading, but it has very few books. When I asked why the centre does not make use of the regional library, the teachers replied: "They will not go to the library. They will end up loitering in the town." In addition, there is a great shortage of textbooks and exercise books. Students are supposed to buy their own stationery but most of them cannot do so. Graduates who have formed a cooperative group buy them exercise books out of the sales from their income generating activities (see below).

Cookery equipment is also inadequate. UNICEF has helped with some cookery equipment, but there are still deficiencies.

To prevent subsequent pregnancies among trainees, there is an UMATI counsellor who visits the centre once a week to counsel girls on family planning. A volunteer nurse visits the centre once a week to educate the girls on childcare and to check the health of them and their children.

Trainees at Matumaini Centre

I interviewed fifteen trainees at Matumaini Youth Centre. One group of teenage mothers who had completed the two-year course and had formed a cooperative group, *ushirika*, and two other groups of trainees who were still completing the two-year course. The group included both primary and secondary school drop-outs.

The centre had a daycare facility with about fifty-three children and three attendants. Half of these were children of the young mothers. The attendants took good care of the children but were not allowed to wash their nappies. The head of the centre told me: "I want the girls to know that although we are helping them they are still responsible for their own children." I noticed that the mothers and their children looked healthy and happy. This was a result of the proper feeding that was provided at the centre. The young mothers took turns in preparing lunch as well as doing the daily cleaning. The cleaning was done in the morning before classes started.

The *ushirika* group engaged in income generating activities such as weaving, and making dolls, handbags, baskets, etc. They used hand looms and thread donated by a lady from Holland. Most of the items were sold at *Nyumba ya Sanaa,* an art and craft shop in Dar es Salaam. After graduating, many trainees preferred joining the cooperative in order to advance themselves in handicraft and dressmaking and to earn some income rather than looking for jobs or starting their own business. After deeper discussions with five of these trainees, I realized that they wanted to remain at the centre since they lacked enough capital to start a small business and they were aware of that it is difficult nowadays to get jobs. Of the twenty trainees who graduated in 1993, twelve joined the cooperative group and thus stayed in a protected environment.

I noted that the young mothers felt comfortable at the centre but wondered how long they would continue to stay there and depend on Sister Ceny San Pedro, who is the head of the centre. She treated the girls like her own daughters. She was committed to instructing them and helping them bring up their children. During an informal talk, one of the young mothers remarked, "I am more comfortable here than I am at home because the head of the centre treats us well. She loves our children and is a very good leader and administrator." I later confirmed this with the teachers, who remarked that the sister was "spoiling" the teenage mothers. Naturally, the girls felt ease at the centre because at home they were regarded as second class citizens. The trainees appeared to like their training programme but complained about the shortages of learning materials and equipment.

I could see that the teenage mothers showed affection for their children and did their very best to take care of them. As I was touring the centre on the first day, I found one of the babies crying at the day carecentre. Suddenly, the mother came running and started soothing

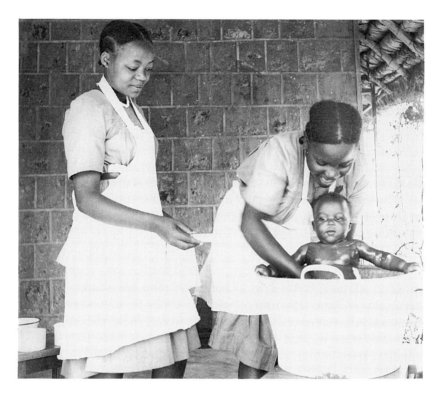

The teenage mothers showed affection for their   (Photo *Daily News*, Dar es Salaam)
children and did their very best to take care of them.

the baby, which soon stopped crying. I also noticed that, sometimes, students fail to be attentative during class, particularly those with children of less than one year. Whenever a child cried, the mother rushed from the class to attend to it without even asking permission from the teacher. At the time of the visit, there were three babies younger than one year.

On the whole, the atmosphere was conducive to learning because of the positive attitude of the head of the centre and the teachers towards the young mothers. The girls were keen to study and seem to be hopeful that the training will enable them to open a small business, such as dressmaking or tailoring, selling bites and snacks, or securing employment so that they can provide for their children and themselves. I observed that the young mothers, in particular the cooperative group, were always singing while cleaning and sewing. Indeed, they were quite noisy, with their laughter and jokes.

Interviews with the teachers

At Matumaini Centre, I interviewed the three permanent teachers and four part-time teachers. The latter also taught at the nearby Lugalo secondary school. This is their account of their views of the girls:

> Most of these teenage mothers are adolescents who are still growing up. Some of them are difficult to manage because they entered adulthood before they were ready for it. Normally, after falling pregnant, the girls become frustrated. Consequently, they sometimes they do not want to listen to their parents. The parents on the other hand get demoralized. They feel that they have lost control over their daughters and decide to disregard them. As a result, some teenage mothers are tempted to look for men in order to have some income.

> When they come to the centre, they get to understand that they have to change their attitude or otherwise they will lose everything in life. At the centre they feel they have a future. Most of them feel guilty about the pregnancy and are ready to reform and complete their training. So far, since we started only two girls have dropped out due to falling pregnant after joining the centre.

> We have noticed that the girls improve in character and develop some confidence after staying at the centre for awhile. Nowadays, they look tidy and dress smartly. One of them will soon get married to the same young Maasai man who made her pregnant. We normally tell them that if they take proper care of themselves and their children, men will be attracted to marry them because they know that the girls will become good housewives, but if they neglect their children nobody will look at them.

> They are happy and proud to have secondary school teachers to teach them. They enjoy working at the school, cleaning the surroundings and growing vegetables in the garden.

Views of the attendants

During a focus group discussion the attendants made the following comments:

> Some of these girls are quite obedient. However, there are a few who are rude even to their teachers. They feel they are mature enough and equal in status because they have children. Some of them cannot follow instruction. For instance, they put their children in the wrong places and the sister has to remove them and put them in the proper place.

> In beginning, some of them were quite obedient. But when their children grew up and after they themselves got used to the centre, they seemed to take the place for granted and forget about their problems.

When these teenage mothers came to the centre, they were in a pathetic condition. Some of them could not afford to buy even body lotion but now they are better off and they can even dress well and look quite pleasant. In the beginning, their children were in a pathetic condition too. Most of them were undernourished. The head of the centre had to provide them with milk and vitamins to enable them to survive.

Those who are in the cooperative group are motivated to work hard since they obtain a monthly income from the items that they make. Moreover, they are paid according to their attendance and the number of items each individual produces. We have observed that they love their children and whenever they get money they buy clothes and other necessities for their children.

According to the girls and the head of the training centre, parents appreciated that their daughters were given opportunity to pursue a training at the youth centre. However, most of them could not afford to make any contribution towards educating their daughters. A small number of about six parents could afford to pay tuition, but were reluctant to do so. They felt that their daughters had misused their opportunity to study so they had no need to worry about them. Some of the parents feel that the sisters obtain a lot of money from the church to train their daughters, and they thought that would suffice.

Mama Clementina Foundation Hostel

The Mama Clementina Foundation (MCF) hostel was opened in 1984. It started by accommodating teenage mothers who fell pregnant at school. The hostel was built on the premises of Weru Weru Secondary School in Moshi. "Mama Clementina" was an Italian nun who worked in Iringa in the 1920s. The founder of the hostel was brought up by the nun. The founder was the headmistress of Weru Weru Secondary School in the 1970s and 1980s.

The main difference between teenage mothers and their fellow students was that the former stayed at the hostel while studying. They were also treated as private candidates and, therefore, had to sit two papers for each subject in their final examinations, which are conducted at Form 4 in the eleventh year of the school.

Funds to run the hostel were obtained from income generating activities such as flour milling, maize and vegetable farming, cattle keeping, and selling snacks. Other sources of finance were the Danish International Development Authority (DANIDA) and the founder of the hostel, who made personal donations in order to sustain it.

Attitudes of teachers and fellow students

I learned from the teachers that despite pregnancy, teenage mothers managed to continue their studies and their performance was not affected. This was due to the positive attitude of the teachers and fellow students, who has great sympathy for the girls. As a result, these adolescent mothers were inspired to continue their education till they completed Form 4/Form 6, equivalent to Grade 12 and Grade 14 respectively.

However, the community near the school was sceptical of the success of the undertaking. They found the idea of allowing unmarried girls who fell pregnant to continue with their education to be absurd and undesirable, whereas the parents of the girls appreciated the efforts that were made by the headmistress of Weru Weru that enabled their daughters to complete their O level and A level education.

Unfortunately, the other teachers at the school had not the same courage or authority to safeguard the MC-hostel. When the founder of the school retired, the hostel was phased out.

Mbeya Youth Centre

The Mbeya Youth Centre, which started operating in 1989, is run by UMATI. Unfortunately, the centre had to be closed in 1991 after the death of its coordinator. It was reopened in September 1994. I was told that Mbeya was chosen as a training centre for youths because the women there are known to be aggressive in business. It was expected that the centre would provide the necessary skills and knowledge to enable the adolescent mothers to start their own business and, therefore, be able to bring up their children. In February 1995 the centre had registered twenty-one teenage mothers.

Funds to run the centre are obtained from the head office of UMATI. A few companies such as Matsushita occasionally give donations to the centre.

When I visited the place, the central building, which is leased, was being renovated. However, construction of the new building in the town centre had already started. The present building has a nursery for children, one classroom, needlework and cookery rooms, two offices, (including one for the coordinator of the centre), a kitchen, store, and toilets.

The Mbeya Youth Centre offers four main subjects: family life education, cookery, needlework, and handicraft. Counselling is provided as a service. The coordinator informed me that he was planning to introduce evening classes in commercial tailoring and carpentry. I also learned that an evaluation of the centre would be made after one year.

The major problem noted was, as usual, the lack of adequate teaching materials and equipment. Teachers complained that they have to buy their own books and sometimes they had to borrow from other schools and colleges. They also needed teaching aids like posters, pictures, charts, and films to make learning more interesting and effective.

Trainees at the Mbeya Youth Centre

I interviewed eight trainees who were in their first year of training. Their ages ranged between 16 to 19 years. Although the small institution had a daycare centre, only three of these adolescent mothers took their children to the centre. A large number of them preferred to leave their children at home with their grandmothers and younger sisters. The children at the centre looked healthy, but needed warm clothes and beddings, since Mbeya is a cold place. The majority of the unmarried mothers looked healthy and at ease. (However, one of my interviewees looked miserable and untidy.)

Three of the eight girls who I interviewed dropped out of school at secondary level while the rest did so at primary level. I noticed that the secondary-level girls were more confident and appeared to be in better spirits compared to the primary school drop-outs. The former were more mature and their parents were more capable of supporting them. However, one of these girls, Neema, stood out from the rest.

I felt sympathetic towards Neema, a 16-year-old girl who fell pregnant in the sixth year of school. I noticed that she was always smiling. During a long talk with her, I learned that she was receiving much support from her parents: "My parents provide most of the basic needs for me and the baby. My mother loves my baby and gives me a lot of support. She takes care of her while I am studying at the centre. They were angry with me when I fell pregnant, but after my delivery they took pity on me on account of my age." Since both parents were working, they could afford to support her.

The girls learned about the training centre through various sources. Some were informed by their relatives while others got the information through their school teachers. The UMATI office in

Mbeya served as a good source of information, in particular the peer counsellors who are involved in the family life education programme. Ward executive officers were another source of information.

The favourite subject among teenage mothers is dressmaking, since most of the girls wanted to become tailors and generate some income. The young mothers had great expectations when they joined this centre. They expected to acquire skills that would enable them to earn some income and at the same time be able to make their own clothes and those of their children. I was impressed by their determination and self-reliant spirit. A trainee, known as Hilda, told me, "I was tired of staying at home so I decided to learn dressmaking", while Susan said, "the certificate which I will obtain will enable me to get a job in a restaurant, canteen or hotel."

The girls were to some extent inspired by those who had completed their training earlier. Hadija mentioned that one of the girls who completed her training visited us recently and informed us that she had opened an embroidery business in Dar es Salaam. She told us that she is making a good profit from the business.

Fifteen of the trainees said that they would like more subjects to be offered in their programme. For example, they would like to learn English so as to be able to communicate with foreigners and read books written in English. They were also interested in bookkeeping and agriculture. Two wanted to learn more about nursing so that they can treat their children when they fall sick because it is becoming very expensive to send them to hospital. Obviously, the teenage mothers are keen to study practical subjects that are useful in their lives.

After delivery these trainees had experienced three major problems: financial constraints, lack of accommodation and housing, and reproductive health problems

Although three-quarters of the parents took care of their daughters's children while they pursued their training, some parents could not afford to cover the basic needs of their grandchildren and daughters and only one of the twenty-one trainees was supported by the father of the child. The girls commented as follows:

– My mother is helping me but she cannot afford to pay the monthly bills for my babymilk. I have to undertake some petty business to pay the bill and buy some of the baby's requirements.
– I take care of myself while studying. In the evening and during the weekends, I have to do some *shamba* work and petty business. I grow maize and beans. I also sell doughnuts (*maandazi*).

- My auntie kicked me out of the house when I fell pregnant, so I decided to go in for some petty business for six months before joining this centre. The money I got enabled me to take care of the baby and myself when I began studying.

Concerning reproductive health problems after delivery, three girls reported:

- I had a serious stomach ache. I got the same problem again this year.
- I often have a backache but I have already seen a doctor.
- I fainted after delivery. The doctor told me that I was anaemic, but now I am fine.

According to the girls, the health problems did not affect their school performance.

Teachers' views

The teachers and the coordinator of the centre informed me that the parents are grateful that their daughters have the opportunity to study at the training centre. The coordinator said:

> Actually, some parents came personally to seek for admission of their daughters. Although half the parents can hardly afford to pay tuition for their daughters they are willing to look after their grandchildren so that their daughters can receive training. To enable teenage mothers to come for training the centre normally provides them with a weekly basis bus fare.

The main problem, according to the teachers was irregular attendance. Of the twenty-one registered trainees, only twelve attended the course regularly. Some of the girls ask permission to take their children to hospital, and by the time they are through it is too late to go to the centre. However, there were a few who stayed at home and pretended that they had taken their children to the hospital. Poor attendance could also be caused by transport difficulties. The amount of money (400 shillings) given to the trainees is not enough for those who live far away from the city centre.

The teachers have mixed feelings. I observed that some teachers were sympathetic to the trainees and appeared to understand their situation while others did not care. The more mature teachers seemed to understand the girls better than the younger women teachers.

Experience and training also contributed to the teachers' empathy and ability to cope with the young mothers. The following views were expressed during a focus group discussion:

> Some of these girls are still in the process of growing up. Sometimes they get confused or lose direction due to peer influence. The teenage mothers are in a difficult position because suddenly they find themselves in an adult situation when they are not ready for it. We have observed that sometimes they lack concentration in the classroom, because of various personal problems for example with accommodation or fatigue as a result off their extra responsibilities in childrearing. The same girls have to perform domestic chores in the home, as their parents still expect for their help.

> We have observed that the girls' behaviour depends on their home background. Some of the girls come from broken homes or are brought up by single parents. Others live near bars or were brought up by parents who own bars or local beer stores. In fact, some of these girls may have fallen pregnant because their parents were so engaged in brewing and selling local beer that they had no time to give guidance or counselling to their daughters. It is also possible that the girls were made pregnant by customers of the family business.

> So far, the young girls have tried to cope with their studies and childrearing. We can see some improvement in their behaviour. At first, they used to fight a lot among themselves but they no longer do that, probably because they are now more familiar with each other. We have also observed that they tend to show some solidarity since they have suffered the same hardships. For instance, they have all experienced neglect by their parents and shame in society.

According to the teachers, the performance of the trainees was satisfactory. About three-quarters of them were interested in studying. Personally, I felt that more effort should be put into creating a more conducive environment for learning. This requires initiative from the head and teachers. Money is also needed to purchase things like desks, cupboards, cabinets, teachers' tables and chairs, and teaching materials, equipment, and indoor games.

The following is an account by four attendants during a focus group discussion:

> Some of these girls are confused. They cannot follow instructions. You tell them to do something but they do it in a different way. They are not obedient either. They are rude and do not know how to be punctual. What annoys us is that no measures are taken to discipline them. The management is not strict with these girls.

They said in Kiswahili *"walimu wanawaharibu kwa kuwabembeleza"* which means the teachers are spoiling them by not being strict. "We feel that most of these girls will benefit from the training but there are about six who are very difficult to discipline. Their attendance is irregular and they are very rude."

Comparison and discussion

Matumaini Youth Centre is managed by a religious group, the Mary-knoll Sisters, while Mbeya Youth Centre is managed by the Family Planning Association of Tanzania (UMATI). This fact alone created some differences. I had the impression that Matumaini Centre had more funds, because it was better of in terms of equipment, material, and personnel compared to Mbeya Youth Centre. Matumaini appears to be better established although it started a year later. Established in 1989, Mbeya Youth Centre was closed after two years. When I visited the centre, it had just resumed operation. A wider variety of subjects is offered at Matumaini, so the young mothers were more satisfied with the training programme compared to their Mbeya counterparts. At Matumaini, there were few primary school drop-outs while at Mbeya it was the reverse. Mbeya Youth Centre provided mainly vocational subjects plus family life education and counselling, while Matumaini Youth Centre also offered school subjects at the secondary level.

It was observed that the first two months were quite difficult for teenage mothers since they had small children to support, household chores to do, and studies to cope with. Yet, step by step, they managed to take control of the situation. I feel that the counselling provided at the centres and the support and commitment of the teachers encouraged adolescent mothers to pursue their training.

The two centres try to inculcate a spirit of self-reliance by involving the girls in income generating activities, cleaning up, and where possible, growing and preparing their food. Matumaini had a bigger plot, so it could grow green vegetables, sweet potatoes, and strawberries. The centre also had a piggery and chicken projects. The products were used to feed the teenage girls and the teachers for lunch. As the Mbeya Youth Centre lacked land, the trainees could not grow anything or run any food projects. However, the girls prepared tea and snacks for their tea break. They also sold snacks in order to generate

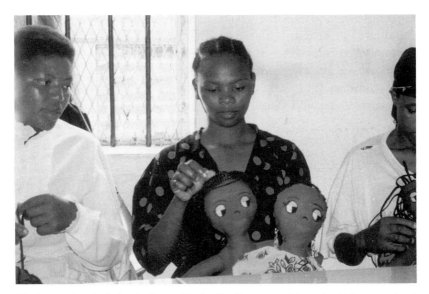

The two centres try to inculcate a spirit of self-reliance   (Photo Alice K. Rugumyamheto)
by involving the girls in income generating activities.

income. These activities were done everyday before the learning sessions started at 8:30 a.m.

The objectives in establishing the two centres were similar: they both aimed at enabling young mothers to complete their education and acquire employment skills. However, at Matumaini Centre there was more emphasis on self-reliance while at Mbeya Youth Centre counselling and knowledge of family life education were more to the forefront.

The two centres for adolescent mothers laid weight on domestic science subjects. This could be due to the common belief that a woman must know how to cook and sew. As we move towards the twenty-first century, it might be timely to include subjects like typing and computer skills, English, agriculture, and commercial subjects in their curriculum.

The trainees at both centres obtained their information about the opportunities for girls who had dropped out due to pregnancy from the same sources: relatives, fellow trainees, friends, primary school teachers, and ward executive officers. The sustainability of the training centres for these young mothers is questionable. It is difficult to run the centres because the parents' contributions are minimal. So far, the centres have not enough capital to start reliable income generating activities. For instance, Matumaini had a small poultry project but kept only sixty chickens.

However, the two centres demonstrate that adolescent mothers can become useful members of society if given the appropriate support, knowledge, and skills. Thus pregnancy is not the end of education.

Reference

Rugumyamheto, A., V. Kainamula and J. Mziray, 1994, "Adolescent Mothers", in Z. Tumba-Masabo, and R. Liljeström (eds.), *Chelewa, Chelewa. The Dilemma of Teenage Girls.* Uppsala: Scandinavian Institute of African Studies.

Chapter 11
Reflections

Magdalena K. Rwebangira

The studies in this book are thoughtprovoking. On the one hand, they show the profound diversity among the different communities of Tanzania, despite the common use of Kiswahili throughout the country. On the other hand, these studies illustrate how a modernization mission from the centre may fail to have its intended impact on community life, despite the good intention of its initiator. The reasons for this failure may be many, as noted in the introductory chapter, "Cultural Conflicts and Ambiguities", but the complexity of local customs is one of them. Without understanding the relevant dynamics of local customs and attitudes, as well as their significance to the people, change initiated from without becomes both ineffective and unsustainable. To effect change in local customs there is a greater need to understand a people's way of life from their point of view and how this differs from that of the modernizing mission.

Moreover, we have been cautioned that generalization can lead to misconceptions about the life of a community and misunderstanding of the diversity of practices in individual families in real life. This became clear from our observation of matrilineal communities where traditionally maternal uncles took care of their sisters' children and such children inherit from them. In practice, some fathers in these communities were taking care of their own children and expected them and not their nephews to be their heirs. The impact of the cash economy and the modernization mission contained in the country's laws is thought to have killed this custom and accelerated the trend away from matrilineality. On the other hand, among the traditionally patrilineal Bahaya of Bukoba and Muleba districts of Kagera region some maternal families were looking after the children of their daughters and granddaughters. So much depends on the circumstances of the child and the disposition and arrangements of individual families. Finally, there is the recognition of the importance and role of the central institutional base in implementing policies and enforcing laws. The absence of an administrative machinery that embraces the whole country renders the law remote from the actual problems of the people. This is not because such laws are irrelevant but because they cannot be realistically applied and uniformly enforced throughout the country. If laws replacing community customs and practices are legislated centrally, they must apply to the centre and the periphery alike.

The message that runs through all the chapters is that we should be alert to one of the major challenges facing our country as we prepare to enter the twenty-first century. This is the challenge of harnessing the creative potential of the youth by giving them the skills and confidence they need to face the future. They need help from the community of grown-ups who should not hinder them but provide positive leadership and guidance to them to achieve their potential as individuals for the good of themselves, their families, their communities, and, therefore, the country. The studies presented in this book do not show that this challenge is being adequately met at the moment. Again and again, we see teenagers being caught up in a transition of social roles and values.

Gender insensitivity

The gender gap in terms of perceptions, obligations, and expectations start quite early. By puberty, boys have developed double standards. They want girls who stay at home to help parents and not to fool around with boys before marriage. But the boys do the opposite of these things and they do them with girls. Where do they expect the desirable girls to come from? Adult men are not free from this insensitive gender anomaly. Throughout the chapters, we see men in different settings cheating if necessary, pledging and urging young women to bear children for them, but in most cases abandoning both the children and the mothers at a late hour. The promised prize of marriage does not often materialize. Girls, likewise, are often naiive and harbour high expectations of finding a husband who is respectful, understanding, and economically self-supporting. It is interesting that the women who earn cash by manual labour are conscious of the need not to add a man as another mouth to feed.

Although the present study does not show how this confusion affects the children, there is evidence that today's Wamwera teenagers

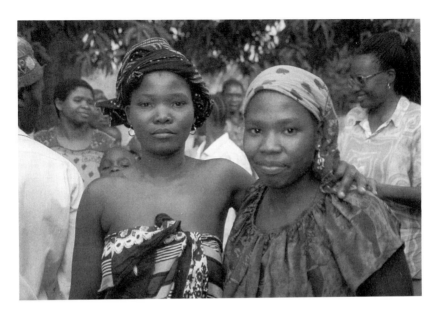

Today's Wamwera girls are less certain of themselves (Photo Rita Liljeström)
than, say their parents, let alone their grandparents.

are less certain of themselves and what is expected of them than, say, their parents, let alone their grandparents. Similarly among the Wagogo and Wayao, we see the rude interruption and disruption of a community's way of life without its replacement by another viable socialization system. While this disruption invariably evokes feelings of resentment in the adult community on the one hand, and on the other, determination to succeed by the modernizing crusader, it is the youth who are caught in the middle. They lack the community knowledge possessed by their parents and faith in the new knowledge preached by the crusaders of the inadequate civilizing mission. Consequently, they are often alienated and confused and reports of stowaway Tanzanian youths caught at sea and repatriated from distant lands or mercilessly drowned have become regular in the media.

Family values

African family values have long been viewed as communal and overly protective of family members, both embracing and elastic, always available to its own. There is a proverb among the Bahaya of

Bukoba in Kagera which states *"emibili tefunda ekifunda eba mitima"*, meaning that the only room too small to physically accommodate human beings is the human spirit. Moreover, strict rules jealously guarded kinship membership through marriage and the affiliation of children. Great significance was placed on marriage, and the pubescent girl was valued primarily for the bridewealth her father or uncle would fetch on her marriage.

Marriage is one of the oldest and strongest of traditional institutions. It is the basis of family life in most legal systems of the world. Marriage also engenders kinship and lineage affiliation. In precapitalist societies, which constitute most rural Tanzanian communities, marriage is part of the basic unit of production. No wonder that marriage is highly regulated. However, some older forms of regulation are giving way to new forms. For example, we have seen how important virginity was among Nyakusa, but exists no more in most of the communities studied. The forms of marriage included kidnapping. Now there is the 1971 *Law of Marriage Act* stipulating that a purported marriage is not legal if, among other things, it involves a minor or is involuntary. In terms of recent amendments to the *Penal Code* under the *Sexual Offences Provision Act*, 1998, such a purported marriage falls within the definition of rape. If consummated, it is punishable by life imprisonment.

Another example is the ranking of wives in polygamous marriages. The first wife in a traditional marriage enjoyed a special status above all the other wives as she was being the manager and custodian of household resources. Today, such a senior wife is often relegated to the village while the husband departs with his junior wife or wives with the proceeds from the sale of the previous season's cash crop to establish a cash-earning business in town.

Old institutions are now changing and changing fast. In the past women married soon after menarche and out-of-wedlock pregnancies were rare. Today education, health concerns, and employment opportunities for women have led to the postponement of marriage. This has contributed to an increase in adolescent pregnancies. Whereas in the past, there was a scarcity of marriageable women, now there are plenty of unmarried women, especially in urban areas where customary restrictions are much looser. The large supply of girls is cited as one of the main reasons why boys refuse to marry, the implication being that sex is for pleasure rather than a sacred socially sanctioned rite inseparable from marriage and procreation.

Sex in marriage not only entails human reproduction but also the attendant norms. The increasing trend towards sex for pleasure tempts men to escape their traditional responsibilities and displace their economic burdens on women. We are witnessing an accelerating erosion of communal obligations and the breakdown of the African family. In the case of adolescents, this burden falls squarely on the shoulders of the girl's parents. What does this say about improving the status of the girl-child in the community? Will the announcement of the birth of a girl be greeted with as much excitement and contentment as that of a baby boy? What has happened to men?

The forces of change

Because the forces of the twentieth century that have had such an impact on the traditional family, such as economic reform and liberalization, there are some fundamental changes taking place. There is a decline in peasant agriculture resulting in a growing crisis in production and reproduction. The existing agricultural system exploits women and youth at the household level. Consequently, women and youth are leaving agriculture to look for alternatives, perhaps paid work and autonomy beyond customary law restrictions, often in urban areas and in budding trade and mining centres. A good number of girls who migrate in this manner are either full-time or part-time prostitutes. On the other hand, there is evidence that women with cash incomes can participate more effectively in decisionmaking at the household level. Thus a major change in the division of labour is taking place. The economic reforms have perhaps hastened this change.

While the decline in male employment and incomes has shifted the burden of providing cash requirements to women, women still do not have better opportunities for employment and incomes-generation in the customary patriarchal setting. Therefore, they have had and will continue to look for unconventional means of earning cash to raise their children, sustain themselves, and reproduce the family. This calls for an urgent development strategy that will reorient people towards the new realities.

One such strategy could be the reallocation of basic productive resources such as land. The monopoly of male elders over land should end. Women and young people, irrespective of gender, also need land in their own right in their villages. A young woman should not have the choice between two evils to either work on her father's (or her brother's) or her husband's land. She should have the option of work-ing for herself on her piece of land if she wants. Marriage should not take away this right but allow her and her spouse to keep open their options of either settling on her land or his. Furthermore, gender-based discrimination in accessing and controlling land is not in our long-term best interests, let alone being in violation of women's human rights to economic and social security. For how can women be expected to support a system that does not support them?

Tanzania is about to reform its land law. The civil society has made several recommendations for the new law, including democrati-zation of land tenure to allow for equitable representation of women and youth on decisionmaking bodies on land matters, such as alloca-tion committees, and land use and dispute settlement forums. Others include divestiture of the ultimate (radical) title in land from the pres-ident, as is the case at present, to an autonomous body accountable to parliament, and the issuance of joint titles to spouses in the titling and registration of land formerly held under customary land tenure. In the case of polygamous marriages, the recommendation is that the title will bear the names of each wife jointly with the husband. Indepen-dent allocation to youths irrespective of gender is another recommen-dation.

Paying heed to the past

Very few people would disagree that there is invaluable wealth in many traditional institutions, such as rites of passage. In one sense they are educational, psychologically empowering, and to some extent establish a strong social support system with practical knowledge for surviving and dealing with known life-threatening situations, such as childbirth. One of the most memorable experiences my husband and I had in Oregon, USA, in the 1980s was participation in Lamanze classes and subsequent the birth of our youngest daughter. Having given birth three times before, I kept wondering why nobody had thought of these classes before! Little did I know that some communities in Tanzania had generations before actually built a similar curriculum into their marital initiation customs for both men and women.

Paying attention to the future

In Tanzania, as elsewhere, teenage girls are, by all indicators, the women of today and the future, the key to tomorrow's sustainable development. In 1995, the number of women between 15 and 49 years was 6.9 million. In 1998, it is 7.5 million, and in 2020 it will be 14.3 million. The rate of increase of this population between 1995 and 2010 will be 56 per cent. Reproduction is interlinked with economics. Holding fathers responsible for their share in the economic burdens of reproduction is an inescapable necessity. The need for an effective machinery to cover all the country and serve all the people cannot be overemphasized. The state's failure to fill this void will remain a major impediment to the achievement of reproductive and sexual health and rights.

Hope is what we need. If the youth is the hope of the future, to give youth hope is to give meaning to our future.

References

Azimio la Uhai, Haki Ardhi. Dar es Salaam.

Kikosi cha kuteka Jinsia katika Ardhi.

"Tanzania's Country Paper on Gender and Law", 1998, in G. Gopal and M. Salim (eds.), *Gender and Law: Eastern Africa Speaks.* Proceedings of the conference organized by the World Bank and the Economic Commission for Africa. Washington DC: The World Bank.

Mbilinyi, M., 1998, "The End of Small Holder Farming". Public lecture organized by the Economic and Social Research Foundation, Dar es Salaam.

Population Reference Bureau, 1998, Washington DC: Media Outreach Publications.

Biographies of the authors

Virginia Bamurange , born 1953 in Cyangungu, Rwanda
M.Sc. (biology) University of Dar es Salaam
M.A. (counselling) University of Reading
Youth Counsellor and Project Leader of the Adolescent Sexual and
Reproductive Health Project at the African Medical Research Foundation
(AMREF)
Member of the Institute of Development Studies Women's Study Group
(IDSWSG) at the University of Dar es Salaam
Member of Young Women Christian Association (YWCA) and Association of
Africa Women for Research and Development (AAWORD)
Mother of two children

Rosalia Sam Katapa, born 1949 in Tukuyu, Mbeya
M.Sc. (mathematics and statistics) University of Carleton
Ph.D. (statistics) University of Toronto
Professor of statistics at the University of Dar es Salaam
Mother of three children

Rita Liljeström, born 1928 in Helsinki, Finland
Professor Emerita in sociology at the Swedish Council for Research
in Humanities and Social Sciences
Mother of three children

Juliana Chediel Mziray, born 1949 in Same, Kilimanjaro
Diploma in office management
Self-employed in business and farming
Researcher at the Institute of Development Studies Women's Study Group
(IDSWSG)
Church Youth Advisor and Sunday School teacher
Mother of four children

Mary Ntukula, born 1956 in Songea
B.A. (sociology and labour law)
M.A. (sociology and manpower planning) at the University
of Dar es Salaam
Administrator at the Embassy of Ireland in Tanzania
Member of the Institute of Development Studies Women's Study Group
(IDSWSG)
Mother of six children

Alice K. Rugumyamheto, born 1948 in Same, Kilimanjaro region
B.A. (education) University of Dar es Salaam
M.A. (education) San José State University, California
Educational Planner/Coordinator at the Educational Planning Department
of the Ministry of Education and Culture
Mother of three children

Magdalena Kamugisha Rwebangira, born 1953 in Bukoba
LL.B. University of Dar es Salaam
Master of Philosophy in Law, University of Zimbabwe
Legal Practitioner with own legal practice
Founding member of the Tanzania Women Lawyer's Association
Member of Women's Research and Documentation Project (WRDP)
Member, Advisory Board of the International Women's Rights Action
Founding member of Women and Law in East Africa (Tanzania) and its
current National Coordinator
Mother of three children

Mary Shuma, born 1953 in Moshi
M.A. (geography)
Coordinator of an Environmental Education Programme for
Tanzania for the World Wildlife Fund (WWF)
Member of Women's Research and Documentation Project (WRDP)
Mother of three children

Zubeida Tumbo-Masabo, born in 1952 in Songea
Ed.D. in Applied Linguistics, Teacher's College, Columbia University
Senior Research Fellow, Institute of Kiswahili Research, University of
Dar es Salaam
Founding member of Women's Research and Documentation Project (WRDP)
Mother of four children